# ULTRAPREVENTION

---

## THE 6-WEEK PLAN THAT WILL MAKE YOU HEALTHY FOR LIFE

MARK HYMAN, M.D.
AND
MARK LIPONIS, M.D.

SCRIBNER

NEW YORK   LONDON   TORONTO   SYDNEY

SCRIBNER
1230 Avenue of the Americas
New York, NY 10020

DISCLAIMER

SCRIBNER and design are trademarks of
Macmillan Library Reference USA, Inc., used under license
by Simon & Schuster, the publisher of this work.

For information about special discounts for bulk purchases,
please contact Simon & Schuster Special Sales:
1-800-456-6798 or business@simonandschuster.com

Designed by Colin Joh
Text set in Bembo

Manufactured in the United States of America

5   7   9   10   8   6

Library of Congress Cataloging-in-Publication Data
Hyman, Mark, 1959–
Ultraprevention : the 6-week plan that will make you healthy for life /
Mark Hyman and Mark Liponis.
p.   cm.
Includes index.
1. Self-Care, Health—Popular works. 2. Health promotion—Popular works.
3. Health—Popular works. I. Liponis, Mark, 1958– II. Title.
RA776.95.H98 2003
613—dc21      2002044794

ISBN 0-7432-2711-5

To my children, Rachel and Misha, who inspire me to ask the right questions; to my mother and father, who always encouraged me to ask why; and to my real teachers, my patients, who have offered me the gift of their trust.

—Mark Hyman

To my wife and best friend, Siobhan, whose continuous support and understanding have been limitless; to my three magnificent children, Timothy, Matthew, and Brenna, who are living proof of grace; to my parents, Charles and Bess, who could not have given me a better start; and to the memory of Ron Richardson, a dear departed friend.

—Mark Liponis

# CONTENTS

# INTRODUCTION

For the last decade both of us have been interested in a new kind of medicine, one with a bias toward keeping patients healthy rather than diagnosing and treating disease.

Years before any affliction can be detected, biochemical imbalances exist in the body that trigger illness. These imbalances are chemical and energetic in origin and are affected by nutrients, genetics, and environment, as well as by thoughts and emotions.

To uncover these imbalances, we pay particular attention to the assessment of five key body functions: nutrition, metabolism, inflammation, detoxification, and oxidative stress (we call impairments of these functions sludge, burnout, heat, waste, and rust).

We have developed a six-week plan that corrects imbalances in these areas through medical treatment and lifestyle changes. The restoration of balance can prevent the development of disease.

We call our plan *ultraprevention*. It is a philosophy of diagnosis and treatment that derives from a scientific study of health. We firmly believe that ultraprevention represents the future of medicine. And we believe that ultraprevention will work for absolutely everyone—whether you are feeling very healthy, or you are feeling very sick, or anywhere in between.

This is because ultraprevention isn't about being sick and then becoming well. It's about being well and staying well. (Of course, if you are sick, ultraprevention can help you regain your health.)

Here's something else we believe: that the current medical model is fraught with dangerous myths—myths that can actually create health problems. And we believe that most people (and, frankly, most doctors) know much less about health than they think, because they have fallen for these myths, such as the idea that (dietary) fat is a four-letter word, or that your genetic makeup is unchangeable.

Why did the two of us become so interested in the myths of modern medicine, and why have we worked so hard to find a system to correct them?

Because we have both been victims of these myths as much as anyone else. In a sense, both of us had to become very ill before we realized how to get better, and how to make others better, too.

## MARK HYMAN'S STORY

My mother and father were free spirits, and we traveled and lived all over the world. Then my parents divorced, and I moved in with my grandparents until my mother remarried and we settled in Toronto. I returned to the United States to attend Cornell University, where I majored in Asian Studies.

Although I'd been interested in Chinese medicine as a career, and became a yoga teacher while an undergraduate, I eventually decided to enter traditional medical school and enrolled at the University of Ottawa, where I also did my internship. However, I never lost my interest in alternative medicine.

After a residency in Santa Rosa, California, where I learned how to be a family doctor in a community practice serving indigents, immigrants, and the disenfranchised, I settled in Orofino, Idaho, in order to start a rural family practice. I longed to become the old-fashioned doctor, caring for my patients from birth to death. Orofino, a rustic logging community, gave me that opportunity. The Clearwater Valley Hospital was on the edge of the largest wilderness area in the lower forty-eight states, and there we took care of everything from delivering babies to dealing with trauma from logging accidents to performing minor surgery.

My patients were unusual. For instance: Franklin, a forty-year-old, four-hundred-pound Nez Percé Indian whose drooping breasts, thin black ponytail, and flushed, hairless cheeks made him indistinguishable from a woman. A drifter, he had left the valley of his ancestors for a modern lifestyle that had rewarded him with obesity, alcoholism, diabetes, and a drug addiction; he was now in my care after swallowing a few bottles of pills and forty-eight cans of beer to cope with a rocky romance.

We pumped Franklin's stomach with a large tube nearly the size of a garden hose in the early predawn hours. Hardened to unappetizing sights, my stomach growled. "I'm hungry," I said to the nurse. Talking around the tube in his mouth, Franklin mumbled, "I'm hungry too."

After three years I'd had enough, and moved to mainland China to develop a clinic whose goal was to connect Eastern and Western medicine. I turned out to be one of its most successful patients. While in Idaho I'd ruptured a disk in my spine and had suffered paralysis, nerve damage, and minor pain. No one had been able to help. But in a Sino-Japanese hospital in Beijing, a Chinese doctor used various techniques including acupuncture, cupping, and Gua Sha, which involves rubbing a herbal tincture over the skin (with an object that feels like an ice scraper) to increase circulation.

Although my American neurologist, neurosurgeon, and rehabilitation surgeons had told me that I would never regain my strength or nerve function, my pain disappeared, my muscles enlarged in size, and my limp disappeared. Many years later, I am still pain-free and able to run, ski, and play ice hockey.

That was my first significant personal experience with alternative treatment. In the meantime, I had moved back to the mountains of western Massachusetts to raise my two children, and to support myself I ended up doing emergency room work in Springfield.

This inner-city job took a serious toll on my psyche and my family; I felt completely overwhelmed. Like many doctors, I believed I wasn't subject to the same sleep requirements as the rest of the human race. I often went for days taking just short naps, working difficult night shifts, eating poorly, and drinking quadruple espressos at eleven at night to survive the next shift. I did this for years, neglecting my body's signals telling me to slow down.

Then, in March 1996, I attended a nutrition conference featuring doctors Dean Ornish, Benjamin Spock, and Neal Barnard. That, combined with my work in the emergency room, where I so often saw people at the end of a long process of disease and dysfunction (often self-inflicted), made it easy for me to renew my interest in nutrition and alternative medicine. I realized I had to change the way I worked. Two weeks later, I was offered the position of co–medical director at Canyon Ranch. I didn't apply for the job, but serendipity landed me in the perfect place at the perfect time.

In the meantime, I developed another health problem. Six years ago I took my kids to summer camp in Maine, and while there became violently ill with some kind of digestive problem. Nothing seemed to help, although I tried everything. The symptoms only grew worse.

Meanwhile, my marriage was falling apart, I was fighting for custody of my kids, and also trying to codirect the Canyon Ranch medical department. My life had become so stressful, and my physical pain so enormous, that I often thought I would have to go on disability. My system was in chaos: my eyes surrounded by rashes, my tongue burning, my muscles aching, and my digestion completely malfunctioning. I was exhausted and miserable.

Eventually I realized I was suffering from one of those diseases for which most conventional doctors have little patience: chronic fatigue syndrome. I was now like so many of those frustrating people who complain endlessly about seemingly unrelated symptoms, who fail to test positive for any diagnosable disease, and who don't fall into the Western medical rubric.

All this went on for more than two years, until my travels took me to a Hawaiian naturopath, whose diagnosis revealed that my system had been poisoned by mercury. A level of 0 to 3 mcg in a twenty-four-hour urine specimen is normal. A case of poisoning begins at 50 mcg/24 hours. My level was 185 mcg/24 hours.

It was never clear how the mercury suffused my system; it may have been from eating too much mercury-saturated fish, or from my dental fillings, or from pollution caused by the heavy coal burning in Beijing. Regardless, I undertook a self-administered program to remove the mercury from my system, using various nutritional supplements including garlic, vitamin C, and fiber, as well as a great deal of hyperthermic therapy, such as sauna treatments.

I also restored a healthier rhythm to my life, with regular patterns of sleeping, waking, eating, resting, and working. My diet changed as I stopped relying on caffeine and sugar to keep me going, and instead started using nutrients and herbal therapies that could heal my digestive system and repair my damaged immune system. Now, when my body talked, I listened.

This journey to health took me from learning about and addressing my body's nutritional biochemistry and cellular biology through a process of psychological and spiritual renewal. It allowed me to heal completely, and gave me the basis from which I now heal others.

Too often patients are given diagnoses that are quick and/or superficial assessments of health. But because I learned firsthand what it's like to suffer from what are called nondiagnosable conditions, I have become much more empathetic and thorough with my own patients.

Today, I wouldn't dream of saying that nothing is wrong, as I was told about my own condition. No longer do I look upon people who come to me with a long list of problems as merely depressed, nor do I dismiss their complaints as psychosomatic just because they have no immediately recognizable diagnosis.

As I look back on the entire experience from beginning to end,

I realize that my poor health offered me an opportunity to learn how to cure both myself and others.

## MARK LIPONIS'S STORY

My education was quite conventional. I attended prep school in Massachusetts and then spent four years at Dartmouth College, where I studied the sciences with a focus on biology and ecology. I vaguely envisioned a career in wildlife biology, but when the time came, an overwhelming desire to help others led me to apply to medical school at the University of Massachusetts, where I was accepted.

Once there I studied by-the-book medicine and, after graduating, became an internist to satisfy my desire to help people. I would like to think that, despite HMOs, insurance companies, and the other bureaucratic impediments of modern medicine, altruism still plays an important role in motivating doctors to enter the profession. I also liked the idea of being a "supergeneralist," able to attend to the entire person, rather than being limited to a single organ system like many specialists.

I met my wife in medical school; she did her residency in Boston, while mine was in the Berkshires, so for three years we commuted to see each other. When we married, we moved to Butte, Montana, where in 1987 we started our practices—my wife's in pediatrics and mine in internal medicine.

Like Mark Hyman, I wanted the experience of being someone's personal doctor—to know him or her from head to toe and to attend to all of that person's health needs. My practice handled the gamut of problems from ingrown toenails to heart attacks, from diabetes to high blood pressure, in an area where there was no regional hospital nearby to treat those patients who stump you. In such a remote location, you can't afford to be stumped.

As a result, I gained a tremendous breadth of experience in treating a wide range of disease, from the simplest to the most critical.

And since much of my practice required such skills, I became board-certified in intensive care.

My practice in Montana also gave rise to my interest in alternative medicine. I became frustrated at seeing the same constellation of problems over and over in my patients: high cholesterol, high blood pressure, too much weight, too little energy. I found myself almost rubber-stamping their medications: a pill for the blood pressure, a pill for the diabetes, a pill for the cholesterol. Inexorably, as time went on they needed more medication, and I disliked contributing to this pharmaceutical treadmill. Eventually my interest changed from prescribing the right medications to trying to get my patients off the medications altogether.

Dr. Andrew Weil spurred my switch to alternative, or integrative, medicine. I had heard him give a lecture while I was in college, and his books *Natural Health, Natural Medicine,* and *Spontaneous Healing* fueled my already kindling curiosity about natural therapies. So in 1992 I began a preventive medicine clinic as an adjunct to my practice, hiring a nurse whose only role was to help my patients thrive without medications.

Soon people were coming in every week, regularly tracking their diets, exercise patterns, stress levels, and so on. We also got them involved in a group exercise program, a sort of support group in sneakers, which consisted of walking three times a week. The results were outstanding—some of my patients lost more than one hundred pounds, including one young man who was so overweight that he had to sleep in a chair because lying down would have caused him to suffocate. Our program had a very high success rate for the many years it was operating.

By 1995 my wife and I were ready to return to the East Coast to be closer to our families, and to put our three children through Lenox, Massachusetts's excellent school system. Like Mark, I first took a job in emergency medicine, but when Canyon Ranch called and asked if I would cover calls in exchange for using the facility, I agreed. They soon offered me full-time work, and shortly thereafter, the job of co–medical director.

Also like Mark, I soon became my own most needy patient. Up until 1996 I had been in good health. I was trim, I exercised frequently, I had no apparent medical conditions. But I did feel a great deal of stress. At the same time as I was starting my job at Canyon Ranch, I was working in three emergency rooms. And we still had our home in Montana, land in Massachusetts where we wanted to build, and a house we were renting. So in addition to putting in more than seventy hours a week of work, I had to worry about two mortgages and a rental.

One early morning, while working an emergency room shift, I spotted blood in my urine. I shuddered: Maybe a kidney stone, I thought, or an infection. But there was no time to check—I was too busy taking care of my patients' health. I finished that shift, went home and slept, and worked almost continuously for the next couple of days, and my urine cleared up, so I assumed the problem was improving; perhaps a cyst had ruptured.

A friend who was a radiologist offered to do a quick ultrasound. The news was bad: a large tumor in my left kidney. I then went in for a whole series of tests—CAT scans, MRIs, ultrasounds, blood work, and so on, until it became clear I had renal cell cancer, and the only option was surgery. There was no radiation or chemotherapy available. I was scared, for myself, but especially for my family.

In the meantime, I wanted to know how someone as informed as I was could have developed such a deadly condition. In response, the doctors asked me two questions. Does kidney cancer run in your family? And, do you smoke? The answer to both was no. The doctors had no other questions to ask, because those were the only two known risk factors for kidney cancer. This was not at all satisfying.

I also wanted to know how long it took for the tumor to grow to such an enormous size. My doctors guessed about eight to ten years. A decade! That's how long it took before the first basic symptom occurred that could identify my cancer. That piece of information was perhaps most frightening of all—to think that something so dangerous had been growing inside of me for so long before it caused any symptom. Who knew what else could be growing inside of me? No one, it seemed.

Now that I knew the facts, I underwent radical kidney surgery, which was an ordeal, but a successful one: A seven-inch tumor was removed, along with the kidney, one adrenal gland, and lymph nodes. My kidney had been almost totally replaced by the tumor. Yet prior to my bloody urine, I hadn't felt or seen a thing, except some minor back pain, which I had attributed to approaching forty.

Having cancer affected my life in profound ways. First, it had a profound influence on my practice. As soon as I could, I read every medical journal and searched every website in order to understand my condition. I soon discovered that over the last two decades incidences of kidney cancer had risen sharply. No one knew why. Yet it seemed obvious that our genes hadn't changed. The only answer seemed to be our environment. And by that I mean the entire environment we occupy—not just the toxins in air and water but also psychological factors, such as stress.

Because several new studies pointed to environmental origins for cancer, lifestyle issues became my focus. Within weeks after my surgery we had sold our house in Montana, I had quit three of my four jobs, my wife cut back on her practice, we moved out of our rental into our not-quite-finished new home, and I improved my diet. Although I thought I had been eating well, I now realized I had been eating too much junk and processed food, and I replaced that with the natural and organically based diet I maintain today.

My interest in nutrition intensified, and I've learned more about it in the last five years than in the previous fifteen. I feel great. My energy level is high, I sleep well, my family life has improved. My whole viewpoint is completely different. Every breath I take I cherish. There is no more awesome feeling in the world, and yet it is something we take for granted.

And I have changed my practice forever. One of the problems of modern medicine is that, unless people are in patently bad health, they tend to think of their baseline situation as normal. I find that many of my patients consider themselves well because they don't know any better. I used to be that way—I had this little nagging pain in my back, and part of me thought, that's how I should feel at thirty-seven. I didn't realize it wasn't right, much less that it was cancer. Most people don't realize how good they really should feel. But if you show them a window on how they could feel, people become motivated to realize their potential.

Whereas once the intensity of the intensive care unit fascinated me, I now focus on preventive medicine. Instead of trying to identify or diagnose a patient's immediate problem, I look at how we can see what might cause a problem many years from now. This means that instead of a few minutes with a patient, I spend as much time as possible asking about diet, exercise, and stress, as well as hopes, fears, and dreams.

This isn't to say that modern medicine is bad. It isn't. It saves lives. It saved mine. But my experience has shown me how it could be better.

Several months after my cancer was diagnosed, Western medicine saved my wife's life, too. Siobhan had become pregnant with twins. But the pregnancy faltered, and only nineteen weeks later one of the babies died. In a twin pregnancy, if one child dies, the surviving fetus and the mother are in danger. Half the doctors we saw advised us to terminate the pregnancy, the other half thought we might have a safe delivery. After a great deal of soul searching, we decided that we were meant to have this child, and should give it a go. But five weeks later Siobhan became very ill and was transported to a high-risk obstetrics unit, where the doctors prepared her for a premature delivery.

During the surgery, Siobhan developed severe bleeding, eventually losing all the blood in her body; she needed a transfusion of some twenty units of blood—the equivalent of her own and that of two other people as well. Meanwhile, our poor baby daughter, born severely premature, had weak lungs. The doctors didn't feel she would survive. Nor were they optimistic about my wife, who had no blood pressure. As I held my dying baby, I watched my wife receive last rites. It felt like the end of the world. There wasn't a sound in that operating room except my agonized sobbing. The baby soon died in my arms. But somehow Siobhan rallied and stabilized, the bleeding was stopped, and she survived. After a few rocky days in intensive care and a lengthy healing process, she recovered fully.

Siobhan's catastrophic illness again highlighted for me both the value of Western medicine and its failure to address the emotional aspects of illness and its impact on healing.

As you can see, each of us has been on both sides of the examination table. But we've become much healthier since our crises, in part because we indeed practice what we preach. Following the rules of ultraprevention has made both of us well today, and we know it will do the same for you, no matter what your medical history.

Recently one of our very overweight patients saw a man his own age, but in remarkable shape, emerge from the sauna. He turned to us and said, "There goes a guy who looks like the inside of me that's just waiting to come out."

This is exactly what we believe. Each of you has a healthy core waiting to emerge, if only you follow the right map. As you will see, ultraprevention is exactly the map you need to find that healthy person inside you.

# PART I

# The Myths of Modern Medicine

The doctor of the future will give no medicine but will interest his patients in the care of the human frame, in diet, and in the cause and prevention of disease.
—Thomas Edison

# THE MODERN MYTHS QUIZ

How knowledgeable are you about today's medicine? Take this test to find out.

1. As a busy professional, you must often eat many meals out that you might otherwise prefer to skip or prepare at home. Tomorrow you have a breakfast date. Because you are starting to pay more attention to your diet, you are determined to order the healthiest breakfast possible. Which of the following would be your best choice?

a. Half a bagel with a tablespoon of jam and a glass of orange juice
b. Instant oatmeal and two slices of whole wheat toast with a small amount of margarine
c. Raisin-bran cereal with a cup of skim milk
d. A mushroom, onion, and pepper omelette

Answer:

If you picked (a) you have been misled by too many ads for low-fat foods. This breakfast has little nutritive value. It is made up almost entirely of empty calories and has a high glycemic index. In other words, its main ingredient is sugar.

Choice (b) sounds good, but it isn't. Processed and instant oatmeal, as well as most breads labeled "whole wheat," are actually surprisingly low in fiber, no matter what the ads on television say. And the addition of the hydrogenated fat in margarine makes this breakfast downright unhealthy—among other problems, consuming such fats can lead to premature aging.

If you chose (c), you are once again falling into the sugar trap. Most commercial raisin-bran cereals have a great deal of added sugar, which probably negates the benefit of the small amount of fiber in the bran.

The correct answer is (d). Despite suffering from a lot of bad publicity, eggs are very low in saturated fat, and do not increase your cholesterol. Organic omega-3 eggs are particularly high in healthful fats, and are an excellent source of protein and folic acid. And as you probably know, the veggies add nutrients that are important for your antioxidant and detoxification systems.

2. You are finally slated to take that physical examination you've been avoiding. But your busy, much-in-demand doctor is always rushed, and you want to remind him to give you that one crucial test that will provide you with an inside track on preventing diseases such as heart attack, stroke, dementia, and some forms of cancer. The test is for levels of:

a. Cholesterol
b. Blood sugar
c. Vitamin E
d. Homocysteine

Answer:
Cholesterol levels (a) alone tell very little about the risks of serious illness; checking the type of cholesterol is much more valuable. Levels of LDL, or bad cholesterol, are important, but now we know there are even good and bad LDL types. And, of course, levels of HDL (the good cholesterol) may be more critical than LDL numbers in many people. Add in your triglyceride levels (which may indicate possible heart disease, brain deterioration, and poten-

tially stroke) and you have a much more telling tale of your risk.

If you picked (b), sorry—by the time your blood sugar has become elevated, the imbalances that lead to diabetes have been progressing for years! There are much more sensitive and earlier ways to detect and prevent this tendency.

Although vitamin E (c) is an extremely important nutrient, it does not act alone but in concert with many other nutrients and antioxidants. Checking your antioxidant system is far more valuable than checking this single antioxidant component; this involves looking at the status of various nutrients in your body, certain levels of antioxidant enzymes and reserves of antioxidant nutrients, as well as the activity of free radicals.

If you chose (d)—correct! More than any other single test, homocysteine correctly identifies the risk of such conditions as heart attack, stroke, and dementia years before the onset of any symptoms. More important, if found to be elevated, homocysteine can be easily lowered using the correct dose of B vitamins such as folic acid, $B_6$, and $B_{12}$. (What is homocysteine? You'll find out on page 42.)

3. Like anyone else who reads the papers regularly, you have become increasingly aware of the dangers in our day-to-day environment. But because it sometimes seems as though everything can be hazardous, it's hard to remember what's really bad for you. This weekend you are going to a friend's country home where you may encounter all of the following. Which is the most common toxin with the potential to become the most serious toxic threat in the United States?

   a. Pesticides
   b. Artificial sweeteners
   c. Radiation
   d. Mercury

Answer:

If you picked (a), sorry—although pesticide exposure can be quite toxic and serious, pesticide residues are unlikely to be the single cause of diseases such as cancer, Alzheimer's, or degenerative ailments.

Same with (b)—artificial sweeteners can have deleterious effects on the brain and nutrition, but they are not as dangerous as other common toxins.

Ditto for (c). Radiation is extremely toxic, but except in high-risk workers (e.g., X-ray technicians, radiologists, nuclear facility workers, et cetera), excessive exposure to background radiation is unlikely to be as common as exposure to . . .

Mercury (d). Toxic levels are now epidemic as a result of eating contaminated fish (especially large predatory marine fish such as tuna, swordfish, and halibut, and coastal shellfish) as well as the prevalence of silver (amalgam) dental fillings containing mercury. Mercury, one of the more toxic substances common to everyday life, has been associated with such conditions as dementia, heart attacks, neuropathy, multiple sclerosis, and congestive heart failure. This means that you are not doing yourself any favors when you eat your friend's special swordfish for lunch.

4. Although you've been able to accomplish many goals in your life, you've always struggled with your weight. No matter how virtuous you seem to be, dietwise you're never able to maintain any long-term weight loss. Your weight just keeps creeping up, maybe three to five pounds per year. The most helpful exercise regime to reach your goal would be:

a. Go to a spa for a week
b. Begin walking thirty minutes three times per week
c. Perform strength-training exercises with weight machines three times per week
d. Chew gum all day long

Answer:

(a) Going to a spa is a great way to jump-start your overall health program. But although you're likely to lose a few pounds in a week, unless you make some meaningful long-term changes and stick with them, a spa week alone won't solve your problem.

Although (b) sounds right, it's not. Walking is relatively good for you, but unless you walk up hills very briskly, the number of calories burned isn't very high.

Strength training (c) is correct; especially focusing on large muscle groups such as the thighs, hips, and buttocks builds the large muscles that are the engine of your metabolism. Building muscle is like adding two cylinders to your car's engine—it will burn more gas even when idling. Strength training has the greatest effect on improving metabolism and will actually help you burn calories while you sleep.

Chewing gum (d) is not as silly as you might think. Chewing gum all day can burn significant calories and can produce weight loss of up to eight to ten pounds per year. But it's not as good as (c), and it might put you at risk for TMJ (temporomandibular joint) syndrome, or pain in the jaw.

5. Today you opened your daily paper and read about another danger from another commonplace activity. By now you've read so many of these stories you don't know what's hazardous and what's hype. Among the following, which is the most perilous?

a. Golfing three times a week
b. Taking antibiotics periodically
c. Sending your clothes to the dry cleaners
d. Talking on your cell phone daily

Answer:

We don't mean to scare you (too much) but the answer is all of the above.

Golf courses (a) are maintained using large amounts of chemicals, which means that while on the greens, your body, as you walk, drive, and putt, must expend energy detoxifying itself. Most adults already have overburdened detoxification systems; repeated exposure to these chemicals can lead to accumulation of these fat-soluble toxins in the body.

Antibiotics (b), although occasionally necessary (and at times even lifesaving), are grossly overprescribed. This has led to extreme antibiotic resistance and superbacteria that aren't killed by any of the known antibiotics. Every course of antibiotics leads to your body being inhabited by more and more resistant organisms, which are tougher and tougher for your antibodies to fend off. Periodic antibiotic use also kills many of the healthy, beneficial bacteria in our bodies that live in harmony with our immune systems.

The dry-cleaning process (c) employs many toxic chemicals that leave a residue on clothes. This may explain the link between socioeconomic status and breast cancer in women.

The electromagnetic fields and radiation levels emitted from most cell phones (d) are above those considered safe by the government. They have been linked to many problems, including high blood pressure and cancer (as well as to more frequent car accidents).

6. You know you're supposed to take your vitamins daily. But you don't do it—and you're armed with a ready excuse if your doctor questions you. Join the crowd. Everyone has a host of excuses. Which of the following is the most valid reason for not taking vitamins?

a. Vitamins have never been shown to be beneficial in scientific studies

b. Recent studies show that vitamin C can clog arteries

c. As a vegetarian I watch what I eat carefully, so I get all my necessary vitamins from food

d. I eat plenty of good food so I don't need to take an additional supplement

e. I eat lightly

Answer:

Statement (a) is simply wrong. Multiple studies have proven the value of several vitamins in the treatment and prevention of a number of disorders. Misleading studies looking at supplementation with single nutrients have erroneously created a myth that taking vitamins is bad for you, or that you can meet all of your nutritional needs through food alone.

Not long ago a highly publicized study supporting (b) appeared in the media—but it did not actually show any clogging of arteries. It talked about a potential, but unproved, thickening of the artery walls in older male smokers. This study was misinterpreted and overpublicized by the media before it could be peer-reviewed or published in any medical journal.

And (c) is also wrong. Vegetarians who do not take supplements cannot get enough vitamin $B_{12}$, since plants do not produce it (and vitamin $B_{12}$ is essential for memory, nerve function, energy metabolism, regulation of homocysteine, red blood cell formation, and much more).

Actually, the opposite of (d) is true. The more people eat, the more vitamins they require. Excessive food intake (calories) is the main cause of oxidative stress and increases the body's antioxidant requirement significantly. (In brief, oxidative stress, which you will read about on pages 145–46, means that you are suffering from free radical damage, which can be compared to our bodies developing too much oxidation, or "rust.")

This means that (e) is correct. Eating less means a lower antioxidant and vitamin requirement. Vitamins and antioxidants are required for the processing of food; less caloric intake means lower vitamin and antioxidant requirements.

7. Although for years you didn't care, recently you've made a real effort to improve your health and you see your doctor for checkups regularly. Now, after improving your blood pressure and your weight, your doctor is telling you to lower your cholesterol level. The best way to do that is to:

a. Start taking a cholesterol-lowering medication, such as Lipitor, Zocor, Mevacor, or Pravachol
b. Increase your exercise by going to the gym and lifting weights with a trainer three days per week
c. Reduce your fat intake: cut down on red meat, butter, and eggs
d. Eat more fat from sources such as walnuts and avocados, eat more eggs, cut out bread, sugar, and pasta

Answer:

Yes, the medications listed in (a) will lower your cholesterol, but they won't change the fundamental reasons why your cholesterol is high, which is a poor diet, hydrogenated fats, insulin resistance, and so on. In other words, for the most part, these drugs are just a temporary fix.

Although strength training (b) is an important form of exercise and can help build up metabolism, it does not have as much of an effect on cholesterol levels as aerobic exercise.

Eating lots of red meat and butter is not necessarily healthful, but eliminating these (c) won't help lower your cholesterol as much as (d).

The best answer is (d). Your body needs these healthy sources of fat. Cutting down on refined carbohydrates will help your cholesterol levels much more than cutting down on fat. Walnuts, by the way, are tremendously helpful in lowering cholesterol.

8. Life is pretty good. You've got a wonderful family and some hard-earned financial security. Now that you've worked so diligently to get where you are, you'd like to make sure you can enjoy life for years to come. Specifically, you'd like your brain to function well past the time that you're supposed to be old and feeble. The best "brain insurance" you can buy right now is:

    a. Cut tuna fish and swordfish from your diet
    b. Reduce your intake of sugar and refined carbohydrates
    c. Drink one glass of red wine daily
    d. Take 1 mg of folic acid daily

Answer:

Once more, all of the above. Fish is supposedly "brain food," but tuna and swordfish (a) are extremely high in mercury, a toxic heavy metal that deposits in the brain and accumulates over long periods of time, causing neurological damage that can lead to further disease.

Sugar and refined carbohydrates (b) can aggravate insulin resistance, a common cause of brain fog and long-term brain injury.

Research shows that red wine in moderation (c) may protect the brain from oxidative stress. But drinking too much reduces any benefit you might be getting.

Folic acid (d) controls levels of homocysteine, which is closely linked to Alzheimer's disease.

9. You're walking on the beach and you stub your toe on a large object in the sand. You uncover it and find that it's an old lamp. You know the rules, so you rub the lamp and out pops a white-coated

genie. However, he's not just any genie; he's the healthcare genie, and because of recent cutbacks from the Genie HMO, he's only allowed to grant one wish instead of the usual three, and it must be from the list below. Your best choice would be:

    a. Protect me from cancer for the rest of my life
    b. Allow me to eat as much as I want and never gain an ounce
    c. Protect me from the dangerous effects of our health care system's errors
    d. Eliminate all stress in my life

Answer:

Although (a) would certainly be nice, the leading cause of death is not cancer but heart disease—you're much more likely to die of a heart attack or stroke than cancer.

And (b) would also be nice, but it's not our weight that leads to disability and disease so much as the amount that we eat. Eating fewer calories reduces oxidative stress, the chief cause of disease.

Adverse effects of our health care system (c) are not only common but often fatal, and add up to the third leading cause of death after cardiovascular disease and cancer. But a better choice would be ...

Stress (d), which plays a major role in disease and disability, and contributes to all of the leading causes of death, from heart disease to stroke to cancer. That is why this is your best health care wish. Stress also causes weight gain, loss of muscle and bone strength, Type 2 diabetes, brain atrophy, and loss of sexual function.

10. (For women only.) You're healthy and you take good care of yourself. But your main concern is breast cancer, because your grandmother died of it. The most important step you can take to reduce your risk of breast cancer is:

a. Eat more broccoli

b. Get on a diligent schedule of monthly breast self-exams

c. See a breast specialist every year and have an annual mammogram

d. Reduce fat in your diet

Answer:

Yes! Broccoli (a), and other members of the brassica family, such as cauliflower, brussels sprouts, cabbage, kale, and bok choy, are important in that they provide an excellent means of preventing breast cancer by assisting your body in the processing and elimination of harmful hormonal or toxic substances.

Unfortunately, there is no good evidence that monthly breast self-exams (b) actually reduce mortality from breast cancer. Monthly exams do not seem to detect breast cancers in a more curable stage than do occasional or periodic exams or annual mammograms.

Although an annual mammogram (c) may be one of the best ways of detecting breast cancer, it in no way prevents or reduces the risk of breast cancer. Mammography is simply a screening test for detection. There is also considerable debate as to whether annual mammograms actually reduce mortality from breast cancer.

Statement (d) is simply wrong. Low-fat diets could potentially increase the risk of breast cancer, particularly if your diet is high in sugar and leads to weight gain. Omega-3 fat from flaxseed and fish, and monounsaturated fats (found in olive oil, avocados, and nuts), reduce the risk of breast cancer, so it's important to include these sources of healthy fat in your diet.

If you answered all of these questions correctly, you are one of the few people in this country who isn't confused by the many myths of modern medicine. You may not even need this book. In fact, you could probably come to Canyon Ranch and help us spread the word.

The rest of you, however, should take this next little quiz. What do all the following statements have in common?

- Tylenol is a safe over-the-counter drug.
- The more you eat, the less vitamins you need.
- Your sex life worsens as you age.
- When you have a sour stomach, you should take antacids.
- Eggs cause heart disease.
- Heart disease is a disease of the heart.
- There's no need to worry about dental fillings.
- Antibiotics are a practical way to deal with infections.
- Vitamin RDAs meet your nutritional needs.
- Chocolate is always bad for you.
- You can't reverse biological aging.
- Disease is genetic.
- A calorie is a calorie.
- Water is a healthful drink.
- Milk is the best source of calcium.
- My lab tests came back okay so I must be healthy.
- Doctors know what they are talking about.

The answer? It's not unlikely that you believe some, if not all, of these statements to be true. But they aren't. They are myths, myths that have been promulgated by the media, by uninformed health care consumers, and, unfortunately, by doctors.

In fact, it's not unlikely that because your doctors believe some of these myths to be reality, they may be damaging your health more than they are promoting it—which is why we often say that what your doctor doesn't know may be killing you.

Not only that, but because your doctor isn't doing the best job of promoting your health, whether you're thirty, forty-five, or seventy years old, you are simply not feeling as good as you could, and should, be.

But you don't know that. This morning you woke up with a small ache in your back, your energy level was a little less than it was a few years ago, your stomach was a bit queasy. You're thinking: This is just what happens when you grow old.

But we're saying: Those little aches, those strange creaking sounds, those small pains—you don't have to have them. That's why we tell our patients that, after they visit us, they will feel as though we've rewound their internal clock, making them feel five, ten, maybe even fifteen years younger.

We promise we can do this for you, too. Once you stop believing in these myths, and you start following our program, your chances of being healthy for the duration of your life will increase dramatically.

The fact is, health care in the United States is not as good as we tend to imagine. Most Americans think our health care is the world's best—and when it comes to certain medical treatments, they're right. We often hear about patients around the world with burns, injuries, or unusual diseases being flown to the United States for emergency treatment of a kind that tops the rest of the world.

That's because our model of medicine is based on acute care—we know how to deal with emergencies better than anyone else. But when it comes to medicine in general, the results are startling. A recent *Journal of the American Medical Association* article reviewed the status of health here and declared: "Of 13 countries in a recent comparison, the United States ranks an average of 12th for 16 available health indicators."

Not only is our system ailing, but the application of this acute care model to chronic illness creates an enormous burden of suffering (in-hospital errors or adverse reactions accounts for 225,000 deaths per year, amounting to the third leading cause of death after heart disease and cancer) and an economic disaster of $77 billion in extra costs resulting from the adverse effects of outpatient care alone.

There are two areas in which to fight this decay in our health. The first is on a national level, and that involves confronting politicians, drug and insurance companies, health maintenance organizations, and the other groups that constitute what we call the medical-pharmaceutical complex. That's a tough fight, and one for which most people don't have the resources, or the stomach. But there's another place where you can take on the health care system: in yourself. You don't have to fall for the myths that are creating an increasingly expensive system that seems to be failing in many ways.

How? First, read Part I, where you will learn to debunk all those myths you believe are truths.

Then move on to Part II, where you will learn the new reality of health and medicine in the twenty-first century. Here we talk about our theory of ultraprevention, a method of thinking, evaluation, and treatment derived from the scientific study of health. Through this system we provide our patients (and now our readers) with a personalized road map to health by addressing and controlling what we consider to be the five most important processes of health management—five forces that are found wherever and whenever we trace an illness back to its roots. The five forces are:

- Malnutrition, or what we call sludge
- Impaired metabolism, or burnout
- Inflammation, or heat
- Impaired detoxification, or waste
- Oxidative stress, or rust

These five forces are the new realities of modern medicine, unlike the myths you must dispel to understand health.

Finally, in Part III, we offer our six-week ultraprevention plan, which will help you live your daily life in a healthy, reality-based manner.

There's an old *Peanuts* cartoon in which Lucy is lecturing her younger brother, Linus, about all sorts of information that makes no sense, such as how a little elm sapling will grow into a mighty oak. Meanwhile, Charlie Brown is watching. He eventually comments that poor Linus is going to have to go to school twice as long as everyone else: First he must unlearn all the nonsense that Lucy has taught him, and then he must learn the truth.

We feel that most of you out there are like Linus. You've been taught countless myths, which you believe as though they were truths. They're not. But unlike Linus, who learned harmless fabrications, you're building up a belief system that could endanger your health. It's time to change, by learning about the seven most common myths of modern medicine.

# MYTH 1: YOUR DOCTOR KNOWS BEST

Joe is one of the nicest guys we've ever met. Starting his career as a plumber, he worked his way up from apprentice to assistant manager until he became a partner in his own regional electrical and plumbing supply business. Along the way Joe developed his share of unhealthy habits, most of which he was able to give up. He was once a two-pack-a-day smoker, but quit five years ago. His routine after work used to include a six-pack as well, but he also gave that up, leaving only soft drinks and desserts as vices.

But over the years Joe's work damaged his knees, which became riddled with arthritis, and he's not as active as he was before he graduated to doing paperwork rather than manual labor. He had gained forty pounds in the past twenty years, most of it in his belly.

At Joe's last checkup, his doctor warned that Joe's blood sugar was high, striking the fear of diabetes into him. (Joe's father had died of complications from diabetes; Joe had cared for his father through his agonizing road to death as he first lost a toe, then a foot, then a leg, and finally his eyesight and kidneys.)

Motivated by the fear of following this path, Joe thought losing some weight was the answer, so he started going to the gym and followed his doctor's dietary recommendations. Because of his hardworking, no-nonsense spirit, Joe threw himself into his new routine.

Only a month after he started working out, however, he developed an aching pain in his back and chest. He tried to continue exercising, but he found himself intensely fatigued and often broke into a cold sweat. When his left arm went numb with shooting pains around his elbow, he rushed to the emergency room; there it took the doctors only minutes to diagnose a serious heart attack, which they were able to treat, recommending, however, that Joe undergo a bypass.

Joe couldn't understand how things had turned so bad just when his business was doing well and he had given up his cigarettes and beer (like many, Joe was inclined to think he might as well have kept up the smoking and drinking).

The answer is that Joe got trapped in a vicious cycle created by the five forces you'll be reading more about in Part II; these forces derailed Joe's natural healing mechanism. A re-creation of Joe's health story might go something like this: Joe's diet had been far too high in refined grains, starches, and processed carbohydrates. In order to keep a steady level of glucose in his bloodstream, Joe's pancreas had to make more and more insulin as time went on. Because of an inherited tendency to become resistant to the effects of insulin, which was magnified by his improper diet, over the years Joe's insulin levels rose even higher. This rise in insulin triggered inflammation (heat) and oxidative stress (rust). His joints became painful and he wasn't able to exercise to lower his insulin levels, nor was his diet helping in that regard.

Finally, he developed mitochondrial dysfunction (burnout), which robbed him of energy and added fuel to the fire of inflammation and oxidative stress. There was no way for his body to overcome these effects, which had been accumulating, growing, and gaining momentum for years.

And yet Joe's doctor never noticed anything until Joe's blood sugar had clearly risen out of the normal range. In retrospect, things were obvious—even ten years ago his blood sugar had been in the very top of the normal range, at 105 (normal is up to 110), and his triglyceride levels fluctuated around 200–250 (ideally, triglyceride levels, which may indicate such problems as heart disease and stroke, should be less than 100). The writing had been on the wall, but nobody had bothered to read it.

To make matters worse, even the attention Joe received after his heart attack was only a Band-Aid treatment that didn't address the roots of the problem themselves. Joe was given a bypass (or brand-new arteries he could then clog up again), and he was put on medications for his heart (beta-blockers) that made him even more tired and sent his blood sugar readings even higher. These treatments were not addressing Joe's key imbalances.

Joe came to see us a year ago, and we were able to design a program that gave him a new level of hope as well as a sense that he had some control over his health destiny. The plan, which helped to remedy his insulin resistance, inflammation, and oxidative stress, was so successful that after a month, Joe had lost twenty pounds and felt more energetic than he had in years. By attacking the underlying problem, Joe began to achieve health for the first time in his adult life.

The field of medicine is complex and is changing rapidly. Every day new data are collected, new research is compiled, new information is published. It's hard to keep up with all this knowledge, especially when much of it can seem contradictory. Salt is good, salt is hazardous; caffeine can damage health, caffeine can benefit health. Who can manage to sift through it all, no less make some sense of it?

No physician can track every change in medicine. But some doctors don't even make an effort. This is due, in part, to a lack of time. But it's also representative of other problems within conventional medicine, a profession whose practices were popularized in the nineteenth century and are often hopelessly out-of-date in the twenty-first.

Although enormous advances are made in medical knowledge every day, many doctors are still regularly treating conditions that have no known cause, such as high blood pressure or rheumatoid arthritis, with medications that often are more damaging than the disease itself. It is not uncommon for physicians to prescribe powerful and toxic drugs that can be more crippling than the arthritis itself, through such side effects as depression, impotence, loss of energy, coughing, stomach ulcers, and internal bleeding.

Too often we meet patients with a terrible cough, and when we ask whether they are taking any medications, they'll tell us they've been taking one of the so-called ACE inhibitors (a class of blood pressure medications) for the last six months.

We then ask how long they've had the cough.

"Six months," they reply. But until we draw attention to that point, they don't make the connection. It doesn't occur to most people that their treatment could be doing them as much harm as their illness.

*Because many doctors are mainly treating symptoms rather than causes, they don't think through each patient's case.*

If you have high blood pressure, they'll give you a high blood pressure pill, instead of trying to figure out why you might have high blood pressure in the first place. They stop at the diagnosis rather than looking at the driving forces in their patients' lives (for more on the problems with diagnoses, see Myth 2). Maybe these patients have dietary deficiencies, or are overly stressed, or have insulin resistance, or have a problem with their kidneys, or aren't drinking enough water, or are already taking a drug that is raising their blood pressure, or are eating too much salt. Regardless, they'll never know, because their doctors aren't asking. And that's a real problem that keeps your doctor from truly knowing best.

Another problem: *medical specialization.*

At its core, conventional medicine is built on the premise of specialization—a trend that began in the early part of the twentieth century and continues to this day.

What this means: If you have a heart problem, you see a cardiologist. If you have a tumor, you go to an oncologist. If you have a blood problem, you consult a hematologist. Today's primary medical model splits the body into many pieces before it's willing to part with a diagnosis. It's almost as if there's a doctor for every inch of you.

To be fair, the details of medicine are so vast that doctors must cope with learning an unbelievable amount of scientific information. That's why it's so challenging to be a medical student or a resident—there's so much you need to know, and so little you actually can know. As a result, physicians want to get their hands around something they can feel comfortable with, a piece of medicine they know is theirs to perform competently.

This phenomenon drives specialization. You realize it's not practical to master everything you should know about general surgery, but you can figure out vascular surgery or ophthalmological surgery. This pattern applies to all branches of medicine, whether it's gastroenterology or oncology or any other subspecialty. Doctors focus on what they need to know so they don't have to think about all the other things they don't. What once might have been on the radar screen is now off.

The narrower your doctor's specialty, the narrower your diagnostic possibilities. This means that if you have chest pains and you visit a cardiologist, you'll probably come away with a diagnosis of mitral valve prolapse, or possibly angina. Take that same chest pain and consult with a gastroenterologist and you'll come away with a diagnosis of heartburn. Bring that chest pain to your orthopedist, and guess what: You've got costochondritis, or an inflamed rib joint. Take the pain to a neurologist, and now you've come down with a pinched nerve in your chest.

(Of course, you can always consult a psychiatrist, and he'll tell you that it's not in your chest at all; it's in your head.)

There's an old adage: If all you have is a hammer, everything looks like a nail. Doctors use what they know and what they have at their disposal to diagnose and treat you. If the hammer is their specialty, then they'll drive as many nails into you as they can.

Which leads us to the next problem: *Medicine lacks an organizing theory.*

Conventional doctors have no underlying philosophy guiding their work. Specialization leads to interests only in a particular field of study rather than the entire human system. So when your cardiologist examines your heart, his attitude toward the rest of your body is similar to that of any specialist. He works only on the heart; he doesn't check the rest of you to see if everything is working within the parameters of any philosophy of health. He just fixes what needs to be fixed and sends you on your way. His model is based on often unrelated, pharmaceutically motivated scientific studies that have no cohesive framework or purpose, a haphazard collection of scientific data that leaves both patient and doctor without an organizing principle around which to think problems through.

What if it turned out your "heart trouble" was related to parts of your body other than your heart? What if it was a problem concerning inflammation in your arteries? Your doctor probably wouldn't know.

Education is partly responsible for this narrow focus—doctors learn their trade through medical school and residency. What they get is a crash course in intensive in-hospital medicine. What they don't get is training in 75 percent of the complaints that doctors most typically see in their offices—those related to nutrition, lack of energy, weight control, sleep, chronic digestive issues, depression, anxiety, and all the other common issues that motivate the average person's visit to an internist.

American medicine is based on a flawed model, one oriented toward acute illness rather than chronic illness. Is there a better country in the world if you need an emergency appendectomy, or if you've been hit by a car? No. But for those of us who just want to stay healthy, conventional Western medicine doesn't work. We don't have an establishment that tells doctors how to keep their patients healthy.

Doctors basically have to learn on their own how to cope with health issues other than emergencies. They know how to treat a gallbladder attack, pneumonia, a gunshot wound. Few know what to do with insomnia (except to prescribe potentially dangerous pills) or weight gain (except to prescribe potentially dangerous pills) or allergies (except to prescribe potentially dangerous pills).

Because doctors are trained to diagnose illness, they're not looking at what could promote health. They're looking only for a particular disease. If you come in feeling ill, they'll find a diagnosis for what's bothering you and follow its treatment by the book. If you have symptoms of arthritis, your doctor will come up with one of fifteen preexisting diagnoses of arthritis, and whether or not the cause can be fixed rather than drugged isn't his concern.

Compounding this is a fourth problem: *Doctors don't have enough time.*

According to a study in the *Journal of the American Medical Association* (January 20, 1999), the average interaction between doctor and patient lasts twenty-three seconds before an interruption. Doctors tend to be distracted, they don't ask about your medical history, and they don't pay attention to all your symptoms—because those symptoms don't always fit into their preconceived definition of a disease. In all likelihood, they've figured out your treatment before you've even finished telling them what's bothering you. They've picked a cure out of their cookbook, and once they have the recipe they don't bother listening anymore—they have too many other patients to see. Both of us used to work in emergency rooms, where doctors routinely made a diagnosis in the first thirty seconds of an examination. Thirty seconds! The patients may have continued talking, but it was pointless because the doctor had already decided on a course of action—right or wrong.

A fifth problem: *Insurance companies reimburse doctors only if they make a diagnosis.*

Insurance is paid when a diagnosis is made. If doctors can't write down a code number for a diagnosis, there's no reimbursement. A recommendation for nutritional changes, or lifestyle management counseling, or grief counseling, or therapy for behavior modification, means no payment.

As a result, there's no enticement to provide or promote wellness. Doctors are motivated to make a thirty-second diagnosis, and then perhaps socialize for another minute or so before a prescription is written or a procedure is scheduled.

In conventional medicine, the sicker a patient, the more the doctor makes. That's why we prefer the old Chinese system, where a doctor is only paid to keep his patients well. If they get sick, the treatment is free.

The sixth problem: *After doctors make their diagnosis, the customary solution is to prescribe a drug—sometimes enough to make your health suffer even more.*

This trend reminds us of the old joke in which a woman uses a sledgehammer to kill a fly on her husband's head. She kills him, too, but rationalizes, "At least I got the fly."

Besides being too willing to give out drugs, such as antibiotics, which become increasingly less effective with overuse, doctors often prescribe medications for a symptom that is most likely being caused by another medication they have already prescribed.

Let's say you're diagnosed with high blood pressure. Without asking any questions about diet, exercise, or other lifestyle issues, your doctor rectifies the situation by putting you on a calcium-channel blocker. But now you come down with terrible heartburn, because the calcium blockers have relaxed the sphincter in your esophagus, allowing stomach acids to flow up into it. (A sphincter is a ringlike muscle that maintains constriction of a body passage.)

Your doctor's solution? He doesn't change the blood pressure medicine. Instead, he gives you an antacid. But now the antacid starts blocking the positive effects of the B vitamins in your diet, so you feel numbness in your hands and feet. When you tell this to your doctor, he puts you on nerve medicine.

And so on, and so on, until your medicine cabinet looks like a pharmacy—which, of course, pleases the pharmaceutical companies. They'd like to think that doctors work for them. Because these large pharmaceutical companies make money only when doctors prescribe their drugs, they do everything they can to make sure that this happens, from supporting medical journals with their ads to having their representatives visit every single doctor's office in the country, where they hand out free samples, buy lunch for the staff, distribute gifts—not just paperweights and pens, but toys for the kids, "seminars" at excellent restaurants, junkets on Caribbean islands. And since doctors are required to continue their medical education, who do you suppose generally sponsors that education? Pharmaceutical companies.

Despite all the medications at their disposal, doctors rarely prescribe well. A 2001 study published in *Archives of Internal Medicine* (vol. 161, pages 53–58) showed that 69 percent of patients at the Harvard-affiliated Brigham and Women's Hospital who were given cholesterol-lowering medicines such as statins were not appropriate candidates for treatment with those drugs, according to the National Cholesterol Education Program guidelines. Conversely, 88 percent of those with heart disease who did qualify for such therapy didn't get prescribed these drugs.

We constantly run into patients who are being mistreated with inappropriate drugs, such as Laura. Slim and attractive, with a loving husband and three wonderful children, Laura nonetheless felt constantly sad. The reason, she told us, was that she had been diagnosed with hypothyroidism (an underactive thyroid). Her doctor had then prescribed a medication called Synthroid, which Laura had now been taking for three years. The doctor had told Laura that the drug was working, because her blood thyroid levels were now normal.

But when we took some tests to check for a different kind of thyroid hormone (the active hormone T3) we found it was very low. This was her real problem. Laura's doctor was giving her a drug for a condition that he was measuring incorrectly. He had thought that if Laura took Synthroid, her body would self-regulate, returning her to health. But it turned out her body wasn't converting the hormone he was giving her into the active hormone she needed; he had missed a metabolic problem.

This anecdote illustrates an important point: The most commonly prescribed medication is not always the right one. For instance, Synthroid requires activation or conversion by the body to the active form of thyroid hormone (T3) the body actually uses. Most people are able to effect this conversion easily (which is why Synthroid doesn't cause problems in most of the population). However, some people, like Laura, can't properly convert Synthroid into the active thyroid hormone. This might be because of a nutrient deficiency (e.g., inadequate selenium) or a hormonal issue (e.g., taking the birth control pill), or for genetic reasons.

The solution is to give a different medication that contains the active thyroid hormone T3 (such as Cytomel, thyrolar, or Armour thyroid).

Why do doctors so rarely prescribe any of the latter? Because they've been taught the myth—handed down from the pharmaceutical companies—that Synthroid is the proper treatment for hypothyroidism. Few physicians explore nutrient deficiencies or other drug effects as possible contributors to low thyroid function.

Actually, there is a pandemic in prescribing habits, and we're not just talking about too much penicillin, but also those third-generation, souped-up, atom-bomb type of antibiotics that could drop a 1,200-pound horse, never mind a bacterium. Doctors do this in part because the drug companies are pushing them so hard. They have drawers full of drug samples, so it's easy to hand the patient the first two days' worth of medication; it's a sure bet to kill the infection, because it will destroy anything. After all, if you want to kill an ant, why use a peashooter when a bazooka is available?

This year, seventy-year-old Cassie showed up in our offices almost doubled over with abdominal pain. Ten days earlier she had eaten some suspicious lobster dip at a restaurant and was convinced this was the cause of her problem. We asked her gastroenterologist for her history; it turned out he was giving her several medicines, including Klonopin (an antianxiety pill to help her relax), dicyclomine (an antispasmodic medication), Prilosec (an acid blocker), and Metamucil (a bulk fiber agent).

Cassie's blood tests were normal, but since she'd once had diverticulitis (a common digestive disorder), he thought that it might be recurring, so he wanted to add Levaquin, an antibiotic, and Flagyl, another antibiotic, to her regime—or six medicines for one upset stomach.

We asked him if he would consider giving Cassie some of what we call probiotics. He had no idea what we meant by this term. We explained: Antibiotics kill unfriendly invaders in your system. That's why they're "anti." Probiotics, on the other hand, are natural substances that are good (or "pro") for your body. These include friendly bacteria such as acidophilus, which are necessary for the health of your intestinal system.

Cassie's doctor reluctantly agreed, but then added that he wanted to give her more drugs and a CAT scan if he didn't see an improvement.

In the meantime, we saw Cassie again and told her to take two acidophilus tablets every two hours; we also made several strict dietary recommendations, and told her to check back with us in twenty-four hours.

The next morning she was feeling so much better that she decided to stop all her medications, except the acidophilus, as well as continue our dietary recommendations. A few days later she was fine.

That lobster dip probably caused her condition; it interfered with her gut flora. She needed something to get her body back on track.

All those pills, however, were having an adverse effect on her body. Prilosec blocks stomach acid and prevents $B_{12}$ absorption, the Klonopin was making her sleepy and depressed, and the dicyclomine can also have cognitive side effects.

This brings us to problem number seven: *HMOs.*

Essentially watchdogs, these health maintenance organizations are more concerned with controlling costs than maintaining health. But who truly believes that cost should be the determining factor in health care? And HMOs make no allowance for preventive treatments. A doctor may suspect his patient has a high level of homocysteine, a potentially dangerous amino acid. But if the HMO won't allow a homocysteine test, the doctor must wait until the patient has a heart attack. Then the HMO will pay for the test so the doctor can see if the patient is at risk for one.

Yet study after study continues to show the role of homocysteine levels in cardiovascular disease; the higher the homocysteine level, the higher the risk of heart attack, stroke, and lack of circulation to the arms and legs. Although homocysteine is a naturally occurring compound, excessive accumulation can damage our blood vessels.

HMOs had the right idea, which was to change the system to emphasize keeping people well rather than attending to them only when sick. But the theory didn't work out in practice. HMOs have created a system of checks and balances so complex that doctors' every move can be scrutinized for deviations from practice guidelines, which has resulted in a huge layer of administrative personnel that has essentially bankrupted the system.

HMOs can maintain the level of administration needed to review charts, look over doctors' shoulders, and count all the beans only by making the margins on care very low. This means that a doctor can perform a serious hernia repair and get paid, say, a maximum of seventy-five dollars for his time. Doctors have found they are working more and making less. But to increase their own profits, HMOs shaved the margins even more—so it just doesn't pay for some doctors to work.

We heard of a doctor in Florida who was so disgusted by the system that he decided to charge a flat fee of $1,500 per year per patient to provide them with good care. He quickly signed up six hundred patients and, last we heard, was doing a fine job, as well as earning enough money to make his practice worthwhile.

As long as we're on the topic of prevention, consider the health risks run by doctors themselves. They tend to be depressed, disenfranchised, burned out, overworked, and to suffer a high rate of substance abuse as well. Statistics show that the number of years doctors spend practicing medicine is decreasing dramatically.

Most doctors, too, are suffering from problems similar to those of their patients: migraines, insulin resistance, hypertension, ulcers, anxiety. At Canyon Ranch, we are seeing an increasing number of doctors who are sicker than their patients.

So why do the HMOs insist on the protocols they do? Because of problem number eight: *Conventional medicine often discounts research that doesn't fit with the prevailing paradigm.*

Back in the late 1960s, Kilmer McCully, a doctor at Harvard Medical School, came up with the theory that levels of homocysteine, not cholesterol, were the most likely trigger for heart disease. For all his efforts, McCully was banished from Harvard; in fact, he and his research were literally laughed at. Only in the last few years has the former laughingstock of Harvard been proven correct—

new research has found that homocysteine levels are one of the best indicators for heart disease. Yet today, despite increasing recognition of the importance of homocysteine, most doctors don't bother to check their patients' levels.

Even further back in history is the story of Dr. Ignaz Semmelweis, a nineteenth-century Hungarian physician and obstetrician who promoted the radical idea that the reason mothers who used midwives to deliver their babies weren't suffering from as much postpartum infection and death as the mothers who didn't was because the midwives routinely washed their hands between deliveries. Semmelweis conducted a study and found that just by dunking his hands in a bleach solution he could reduce the rate of death from childbirth by more than half.

But when he proposed this to the medical community, horrified doctors ridiculed him because they couldn't accept the idea that they were killing their patients with their own germ-ridden hands. Humiliated, Semmelweis was forced to leave Vienna for his native Hungary, and it took many more years for the idea to be fully accepted.

Perhaps the most common place where we see doctors missing the boat is irritable bowel syndrome, from which more than 60 million Americans suffer. Irritable bowel syndrome is a disturbance of the intestinal function, with two or three of the following features: abdominal pain that is relieved with defecation; abdominal pain that is associated with frequency of bowel movements, constipation, or diarrhea; and loose, watery, or pelletlike stool.

Today's prevailing thesis is that irritable bowel syndrome is an unknown condition requiring medication to stop its symptoms. That's certainly what most doctors will tell you if you ask.

We think, however, that irritable bowel syndrome is caused by an imbalance of the ecology of the intestinal tract. Like any ecosystem, your intestine—which breaks down, digests, and absorbs food, as well as helping to control water balance and eliminate waste—

contains a delicate balance of living organisms, known as your gut flora. Around 100 quadrillion organisms live within every human digestive tract, which, at three pounds, could be considered the largest internal organ other than the liver.

The healthy bacteria in your intestine, including lactobacillus, bifidobacteria, and *E. coli* (not the killer *E. coli* you hear about in the media), aid your digestion primarily by breaking down tough fiber. These beneficial bacteria also perform chemical transformations such as synthesizing vitamins and nutrients—for example, they manufacture vitamin K and many of the B vitamins. They also digest foods such as flaxseed and soy, and change them into molecules possessing anticancer properties.

These bacteria have an excellent symbiotic relationship with us. They thrive because we feed them, and we benefit from their helping us digest food and produce important nutrients that we absorb into our bodies.

These bacteria also serve another function: They crowd out other, nastier flora in the gut. Because of the stress we put on our bodies through antibiotics, alcohol, sugar, and bad food or water, we often disturb the normal ecological balance in our gut, causing certain bacteria and yeasts to grow unchecked. This creates a little fermentation factory, similar to what happens when you let apple cider stay in the refrigerator too long and the container explodes.

In our bodies, the internal fermentation process causes bloating, gas, and pain. Food remains undigested, and in turn also ferments. When this happens, your breath contains an excess amount of hydrogen, produced from the fermenting bacteria.

Furthermore, the only thing separating us from these unfriendly bacteria is a membrane just one cell thick: the intestinal epithelium, or the gut lining. If just a few of these nasty bacteria cross that lining, they can cause something as lethal as peritonitis, or something as common as irritable bowel syndrome, or even autoimmune or other inflammatory diseases.

The bacteria we like so much aren't interested in getting across that lining, but when the lining is inflamed or injured in some way, more dangerous bacteria can leak through it.

So our guts are the scene of a constant ecological struggle among bacteria. The fewer good bacteria living inside of us, the more likely the bad bacteria or other organisms will have no competitors and will grow and reproduce.

The most common reason for the death of good bacteria is antibiotic use. An antibiotic will kill the sensitive bacteria, and all the ones that are resistant to it will have no competition in the ecological system and can proliferate. In response to rampant overprescribing, the Centers for Disease Control recently issued a plea to doctors to stop prescribing unnecessary antibiotics.

One of the problems that can develop from doctors' belief that they always know best is what Dr. James S. Goodwin of the University of New Mexico Medical School calls "the tomato effect." For years the tomato, which originated in the New World, was a dietary staple in the Old World. But they weren't consumed in the Americas, where they are indigenous, because North Americans felt that the tomato, part of the nightshade family, was poisonous. Not until the 1800s did Americans start to eat the tomato, now one of the country's largest commercial crops.

Likewise, many excellent treatments have been ignored by the medical community for long periods of time, even in the face of their efficacy—just as colonial Americans weren't persuaded by the fact that their European counterparts were hardly dying from eating tomatoes.

Among these treatments, writes Goodwin, is colchicine, a plant used to treat gout back in the fifth century A.D. Once it fell out of favor, it took centuries to return to practice. Another is gold, which, injected in liquid form into the bloodstream, was a popular and effective treatment for rheumatoid arthritis until the 1940s, when it lost favor and nearly disappeared from medical textbooks. Gold has only recently returned to favor, despite the fact that no one knows exactly why it works (which is one reason why it fell out of fashion).

Today countless efficacious treatments are being ignored just as colchicine and gold were for so many years. Not that doctors are trying to ignore new research. They just don't have the time to keep current, and are not taught, much less encouraged, to think out of the box. Instead, doctors are trained to discard or ignore therapies and approaches that have not been proven beyond a reasonable doubt, even if these therapies or approaches make sense from the context of what is known about a particular condition or disease.

So the problem is not just that doctors don't always know best— sometimes it's that they simply don't know where to look. Do you know the old story about the man looking for his car keys under the lamppost? When a friend asks him where he lost his keys, he points to a sidewalk across the street. "Then why are you looking for them under the lamp?" the friend asks. "The light's better here," the man says.

Doctors, too, tend to treat based on where they think the light is good (or, what they know). They don't like to venture into areas where they can't see clearly. So they fit someone with a problem into the existing paradigm. Instead, if doctors (and patients) keep an open mind, as well as continue to learn and grow, we're all likely to stay healthy.

# MYTH 2: IF YOU HAVE A DIAGNOSIS, YOU KNOW WHAT'S WRONG WITH YOU

When Jerry first came into our office accompanied by his wife, Dorothy, they both claimed to know the issue at hand. A former corporate lawyer who had retired to do volunteer work, Jerry was only sixty-eight, but his mind was faltering. Dorothy was deeply concerned about him, as their doctor had spoken that frightening word: *Alzheimer's*.

Dorothy had come along because she feared that Jerry's mind wasn't up to hearing, comprehending, and, above all, remembering. Both of them wanted to know if there was anything they could do about his Alzheimer's, and they were curious about the symptoms they could expect Jerry to suffer.

The conversation was difficult because Jerry truly was addled. When asked about his health, he sometimes couldn't remember what was wrong with him, or even why he was sitting in our office. (Jerry was currently taking Aricept, which is used for Alzheimer's but has not been shown to slow the progression of the disease at all.)

But as Jerry was fumbling around, trying to focus, we were beginning to wonder. To us, the most curious part of his story was Jerry's comment that he had many fillings in his teeth and that he frequently consumed the type of fish most often contaminated with mercury. This made us speculate that, despite the diagnosis, Jerry might not have Alzheimer's at all. He might be suffering from mercury poisoning.

When we measured his blood for mercury levels, we indeed discovered Jerry had the highest levels of anyone we'd ever tested. We went forward with our treatment (which required intensive mercury-elimination therapy). Within six months, Jerry's mercury levels had dropped significantly and his mental functioning had improved.

Jerry and Dorothy were convinced that because Jerry had been diagnosed with Alzheimer's disease, he was going be sick for the rest of his life. But here's something you must remember for the rest of your life: Just because you've been told you have a certain disease doesn't mean you know the cause.

What do we mean by the word *diagnosis*? It's that moment when doctors name the disease they think you have. But having a diagnosis doesn't mean you know what's wrong. You just know what a doctor calls your symptom. You have the name of a disease.

So many times a patient has told us that she has been told she has a certain disease, and stops thinking about it. This happened the other day when a woman came into our office and said she had colitis. We asked her about her symptoms.

She had a long history of trouble gaining weight, trouble with her menstrual periods, irritable bowel syndrome, and, recently, severe canker sores. After a long course of antibiotics for a strange form of acne, she also developed severe abdominal pain and bloody diarrhea, was told she had colitis, and was put on intravenous steroids and other immune-suppressing drugs.

When we asked about any unusual reactions to food, she said, "Yes, whenever I eat bread or wheat or drink beer, I sneeze and get a stomachache."

It turned out she had had a severe allergy to gluten, the protein in wheat, that was causing all her symptoms. Her "colitis" went away when she cut out gluten from her diet.

Or, let's say your doctor tells you that you have asthma. You think you know what's ailing you. But that may not be the case. "Asthma" is just your doctor's way of coming up with a name for your collection of symptoms. The actual cause of your ill health can be any number of things: Maybe you're allergic to dairy foods; maybe you're breathing in toxic chemicals; maybe you're suffering from a reaction to tartrazine from the dye in your chewing gum.

Those are all possible causes of symptoms that might resemble asthma. The name *asthma* itself is just a semantic tool; it doesn't tell you anything about the cause or the source of your symptoms. A better name for asthma, for instance, might be infectious-allergic-environmental-chemical-hypersensitivity/bronchospastic-inflammatory pneumonitis. But that's a tongue twister.

Why is it so important to debunk this particular myth? Because traditionally, once your symptoms have been given a diagnosis, the thought process stops. Neither you nor your doctor have to think anymore. He looks in the recipe book to find a treatment for your disease and tells you what you should do; you, in turn, take a drug that suppresses your symptoms.

We think that the moment you receive a diagnosis is when the thought process should start. Doctors should begin asking themselves: Why does this person have asthma? Why is this person depressed? Is there something causing this collection of symptoms that we can target?

The differential diagnosis, or the diagnosis that tells the patient in a few words what is wrong, is the equivalent of the Holy Grail in Western medicine. When the doctor makes that diagnosis, the doctor is king. It's like winning a game of medical *Jeopardy*.

The real story is that the doctor is not the king. No one can dig right to the root of every disease. Maybe what's really wrong is something your mother ate while she was pregnant with you, or maybe it's the result of interacting with a dog when you were a child, or maybe you inherited the quirky genes of your father.

What must be identified are the interrelationships between a given condition and a variety of other factors and conditions. Asthma is related to digestive health, which is related to liver function, which is related to brain chemistry. Our bodies operate like an old Rube Goldberg contraption in which moving one little lever in one location causes another to move, then another, and soon every other piece of the machinery is in motion.

For instance, the disease known as hypercholesterolemia (a high level of cholesterol) is often considered a likely cause of heart problems. But we believe that heart disease is a multifactorial problem, arising from such issues as inflammation, insulin resistance, oxidative stress, high levels of homocysteine (from a functional deficiency of B vitamins), occult infection (such as bad teeth or gum disease), depression, and/or stress. So when you're labeled as having hypercholesterolemia, you're liable to believe that you know your problem, and it's a simple one. Not true.

The difference between a diagnosis and its actual symptoms is similar to the variance between the current practice of medicine, which is disease-centered, and our model of medicine, which is patient-centered. We feel that, rather than just try to make a diagnosis, or assign a name on which to blame someone's symptoms, doctors should try to identify and understand the factors that led to the development of symptoms or illness in each individual.

Take the case of Rose, a thirty-four-year-old stockbroker and mother of a young girl. Years ago she had been diagnosed with asthma and was treated with the usual asthma medications, including two inhalers, a pill called Singulair, and an occasional course of steroids if she had a flare-up.

Aside from her asthma, Rose considered herself healthy; we met her only because she wanted to take a bone density test, as a friend had been telling her she should try one. Her results did show some bone loss, which is not uncommon in asthma sufferers, especially after receiving steroid treatments, which can cause thinning of the bones.

But we also discussed Rose's history. Rose suffered from severe allergies as a child, as well as frequent bouts of eczema, which eventually faded. Then, in her twenties, she developed asthma along with occasional sinus infections, for which she was usually treated with a course of antibiotics.

Rose admitted that she also experienced frequent digestive problems, which she'd had for so long that she assumed such pains were normal, although she felt her symptoms might be worsening.

We felt that all this added up to more than just asthma. We determined that Rose had an almost lifelong condition that explained not only her asthma but her eczema, sinus infections, and digestive symptoms as well. Subsequent testing confirmed our suspicion: Rose suffered from a strong dairy allergy. When she was a child, this manifested itself as eczema; as a young adult she developed the sinus infections.

Antibiotic treatment aggravated Rose's digestive problems by changing the delicate balance of bacteria in her gut. And as she continued to eat dairy products, her symptoms became worse and the asthma appeared. Now she was taking the standard asthma treatment, which seemed to be helping, but was causing measurable bone loss.

The solution was simple. We eliminated dairy products entirely from Rose's diet. She was amazed at the results. Not only did her asthma improve to the point where she no longer needed to take her medications on a daily basis, but her digestive symptoms cleared up as well.

For the last eighteen months, Rose has not had a single cold or sinus infection. The icing on the cake is that she discovered that her daughter's own skin rashes and constipation were also due to a dairy allergy. Thankfully, her daughter won't have to wait thirty years to feel better.

★   ★   ★

The origin of the name-that-disease myth stems from the basic Western medical model, which arose many eons ago with the first primitive levels of medicine. Here a doctor was called in to see a patient when he was clutching his chest, or when he banged his head, or when he had a tumor growing out of his body. In other words, when something was very wrong, the doctor was supposed to make it right again.

Of course, for many centuries a doctor might diagnose just about anything from devil infestation to an inopportune phase of the moon. Cures were equally implausible, including bloodletting, leeches, trephination (boring holes in the skull), and amputations, all without anesthesia.

It wasn't until after the microscope was invented (somewhere between 1590 and 1608) that nineteenth-century French chemist Louis Pasteur (1822–1895) was able to develop the microscopic germ theory of infection. Through Pasteur's research on infectious diseases such as rabies, anthrax, and chicken cholera, science developed the idea that illnesses were caused by specific germs. Pasteur was also one of the first scientists to show that inoculation could prevent illness after exposure to some of these germs.

The pace of research quickened, and penicillin and other antibiotics were discovered in 1929. Still more antibiotics followed, and by the 1940s there were cures for many of the contagious diseases that were some of the major killers of that time, such as tuberculosis, syphilis, and pneumonia.

With the discovery of germs, medicine possessed an external, scientifically based cause of disease. People were no longer sick from within, but were being attacked by an external factor over which they had no control. We were lucky if we didn't get it, and we were unlucky if we did. The idea that the risk could be managed wasn't a popular one.

Out of this model arose the idea that diseases are things that can be seen (like bacteria), and then labeled. You are sick because something has possessed you, and that something is called asthma, or depression, or cancer.

As Western science advanced this theory, as it became able to cure more and more previously lethal diseases, it also developed the notion that we should attack all illness as though there were a magic bullet for each one, as penicillin was for syphilis.

This led to a frenzied chase for the ultimate panacea, a pursuit that still shapes the direction of our research and fuels the massive growth of the pharmaceutical industry. Practitioners of conventional medicine feel they can find an external cure, that there is one perfect drug for each problem.

This theory can indeed work for some diseases, particularly the infectious ones. But as medical science has learned over time, the more antibiotics we develop and use, the tougher and more resistant bacteria becomes. It's an ever more complex game of trying to be smarter than the germs, and the jury is still out on who will win in the end—the germs or us.

The germ theory also misses a key phenomenon, which is that the host, or what French professor Claude Bernard called the "biological terrain"—our being—was equally as important, if not more so, in determining who got sick and how the illness progressed. While Pasteur championed the attack on the germs, in 1865 Bernard professed that "the microbe is nothing, the terrain is everything." Medical legend holds that on his deathbed, Pasteur said, "The terrain is all," but his revelation was passed off as the raving of a terminally ill man.

The second major philosophical event that helped create and solidify the mechanistic theory of medicine was the work of Moravian botanist Gregor Mendel, the Augustinian monk who discovered genetics through his work with pea plants. By breeding his plants to develop certain characteristics, Mendel discovered that he could then predict the characteristics of their progeny based on breeding patterns.

Mendel's work has, however, led to certain assumptions about inheritance that may be true for certain traits in pea plants, but are not always true with more complex patterns of inheritance in humans.

Science still assumes that, for the most part, our genetic inheritance works like Mendel's pea plants; some characteristics, such as eye or hair color, gender, and skin color, don't change. This gives the impression that genes themselves are unchanging, fixed entities.

But many genetically influenced traits are much less deterministic, much more plastic and pliable. Characteristics such as height, intelligence, artistic or musical talent, memory, muscle fiber type, and lung capacity may have a genetic foundation, but many such traits are also affected by the circumstances of one's environment, diet, habits, childhood, growth, and development.

These environmental factors explain differences in appearance, skills, and personalities of identical twins, who share an identical set of genes. Likewise, our health is not genetically determined. There may be genetic tendencies toward common conditions such as cardiovascular disease, cancer, arthritis, Alzheimer's disease, diabetes, allergies, and emphysema, but these tendencies must be activated by a certain environment, by certain habits, stresses, behaviors, and activities.

The difference between a genetically deterministic condition and a genetically variable condition depends on the number of genes involved. Only a handful of rare disorders, such as cystic fibrosis and Tay-Sachs, are known to be caused by a mutation in a single gene. In these conditions, the gene involved is responsible for a specific and critical enzyme or protein that is necessary for a particular process to occur in the body; if this enzyme or protein is absent or dysfunctional, then a specific condition results.

In the majority of human illnesses, however, and specifically for all of the most common disorders, no single gene is responsible or defective. In these conditions, many genes are responsible, and the expression of those genes is affected by the environment in which the genes reside. So although genes may play a role in these common disorders, whether a genetic tendency is expressed, and how, is highly variable, depending on less predictable outside factors.

The principle here is that the same disease may have ten different causes, or the same initiating factor can create ten different diseases. Modern medicine tends to ignore this. But a condition such as heart disease can be caused by high blood pressure, high cholesterol, an infection, high homocysteine levels, too much insulin, eating the wrong kind of fat, and so on. And then again, high homocysteine doesn't always cause a heart attack; sometimes it causes dementia, or birth defects, or stroke, or cancer. And dementia, too, may have many different causes, as do birth defects, and stroke, and so on and so on.

The more important factor in disease is the person. Certainly there are some microorganisms that will make everyone sick, such as measles. But even in these cases, not every child comes down with measles the same way—if the child is healthy, eats well, and exercises, her symptoms may not be as bad as those of a malnourished, unhealthy child. It's the combination of the virus and you that determines the course of the illness.

Diseases are not independent objects that have a life outside of you. You don't walk into a room and get cancer or heart disease. Don't blame the name. The diagnosis is just the name of the illness. Depression, for instance, is the name of a collection of symptoms such as poor sleeping habits, weight gain, sadness, despair, and low sex drive—but those symptoms may be caused by many things, including vitamin $B_{12}$ deficiency, sleep apnea, poor circulation, psychological trauma, and so on.

Illness is not a random event. It's based on a series of interlocking factors, as we told fifty-two-year-old Martha, who has been visiting Canyon Ranch for several years.

Martha recently came down with Parkinson's disease, which was common in her family. Her doctor told her that once she was diagnosed with the disease, she would have to live with the symptoms it caused, and he prescribed two medications, Sinemet (L-dopa) and Amantadine.

When we met with Martha, we told her that her doctor may have been giving her appropriate treatment, but there were still many unanswered questions. Why had she developed symptoms like those of Parkinson's? Was there anything else we could do to address these possible causes? The only way to know would be through tests.

Parkinson's disease can sometimes be caused by a toxic exposure that damages a certain area of the brain (the *substantia nigra,* or black substance), as well as causing inflammation in the brain and free radical damage (for more on free radicals, see pages 145 and 194). Martha also had a lot of rancid fat in her blood, from free radicals in her system.

Through testing, we also found that although Martha might have been genetically predisposed to Parkinson's, there was another culprit. More telling was her hair analysis, in which we found a great deal of lead and mercury, both of which can be associated with Parkinson's.

Martha's diet was heavily dependent on fish, and this was how she was absorbing her mercury. The lead may have been coming from some pipes in her beautiful but old Victorian home.

(Keep in mind that today we are exposed to more than 75,000 chemicals, many of which are recent inventions. Human systems never had to deal with them before. And simply put, some people cope better than others. For this reason, farmers have a higher rate of Parkinson's disease than the general population, because they are exposed to more industrial chemicals, such as pesticides. Likewise, anyone with weakness in his or her detoxification system will suffer more illness.)

We gave Martha free radical quenchers to lock up those free radicals, told her how to change her diet and increase her exercise, and started her on a mercury reduction program. A month later, her tremors were gone, she could swim and walk freely, and she stopped taking her Parkinson's medication (which we didn't tell her to do).

Martha's doctor guessed that she had Parkinson's—but that wasn't what had been making her sick. Like Jerry, Martha was being poisoned by toxins in her environment, and the inflammation and oxidative stress that resulted.

Remember: Many conditions that suggest distinct diagnoses are more complex. For instance, when someone has diabetes, he or she may also come down with conditions such as high blood pressure, high cholesterol, cataracts, arthritis, or osteoporosis.

Most traditional doctors would consider those six different diagnoses, which by chance could be attributed to this one individual. But they're all connected by common threads, and each can result from the same cause.

Few of us accumulate one condition or disease at a time as though we were collecting shells by the ocean. Illnesses tend to be related. Diabetes is not at base the illness; the issue is that the patient has insulin resistance, inflammation, oxidative stress, or poor clearance of homocysteine from the system—in other words, he or she suffers from one of the five forces of illness that form the basis of ultraprevention, which you will read about in Part II.

Sometimes, when diagnosed with a disease, people alter their lifestyle—and it's often for the worse. For example, Joey, a young Massachusetts police officer, recently completed his training and took a job in a small community police department—his lifetime dream. But before he was offered the job, Joey had to pass a physical, which he felt would be no problem, as he had always been fit and healthy.

And indeed Joey checked out perfectly—with two exceptions. His blood pressure was borderline for his age, at 138/88. But his doctor guessed this might have resulted from nervousness, and said he would keep watching it.

The second problem turned out to be more urgent—Jerry had hypercholesterolemia. His cholesterol level was 248. His doctor told him if he didn't get this down by at least thirty points, he would have to go on medication, probably for the rest of his life. Here's where the battle started.

Determined not to take the medications, Joey asked his doctor if he could lower his cholesterol some other way. The answer was twofold: exercise more and avoid fat.

Since Joey was already running half marathons and working out six days a week, he worked on the fat part of the equation. He wouldn't eat anything with more than a gram of fat in it. He stayed on his diet to the letter and went back to his doctor's office three months later full of confidence. But when the results came back Joey felt as though he'd been sucker punched. His cholesterol reading had jumped to 266.

His doctor said it was time for medications, but Joey begged for one last chance, thinking he might have been taking in small amounts of fats from prepared foods. He was determined not to go on medications. But he felt hopeless.

It was just a coincidence that we met Joey after he attended a lecture at Canyon Ranch during a weekend with his fiancée. Joey was shocked to hear that he was doing it all wrong. But now his eyes were wide open. He increased his fat intake to eighty grams a day of *healthful* fat, snacking on nuts and guacamole, eating eggs for breakfast, and adding extra virgin olive oil to his salads.

Eight weeks later Joey nervously returned to his doctor for another cholesterol test. When his doctor called with his results,

Joey held his breath, half expecting bad news and a prescription, but instead his doctor said, "Congratulations! Your cholesterol is down to 198! Keep up the good work!"

Joey called immediately to pass on the good news and to thank us. He did not have high cholesterol. He was simply malnourished; he had been spoon-fed the myth that fat is forbidden and he had swallowed it. (For more on why fat can be the answer to your prayers, see page 122.)

Another classic occasion for misdiagnosis is menopause. If a doctor determines that a woman is going through menopause, the treatment offered is fashioned around her symptoms rather than the person herself. Her health history (which we feel is critical in arriving at the best treatment) is typically ignored, or at least minimized.

Wendy is a fifty-year-old elementary school teacher who told us of a long history of hormonal problems. She started getting her period at age eleven and was already fully developed in fifth grade, before many of the girls in her class even had training bras. Wendy remembers years of difficult periods, with severe cramping and heavy bleeding that sometimes lasted more than a week.

Wendy's doctor put her on birth control pills to regulate her cycles just before her fourteenth birthday, and she continued to take some form of the pill through college. Only when she was married did she stop taking it, because she wanted to get pregnant.

Unfortunately, it wasn't that easy. Wendy spent four years in fertility treatments, taking all manner of hormone shots and pills, and still wasn't able to conceive. Finally she and her husband decided to adopt a baby girl from China.

But as Wendy proceeded down the road to menopause, when hormonal chaos supposedly leads to stability, her health worsened. She began having extremely heavy bleeding, which her doctor correctly diagnosed as a fibroid in the uterus. She also began experiencing tremendous mood swings, as well as recurring hot flashes, night sweats, breast soreness, headaches, and sleeplessness. More disturbing to Wendy, she started losing patience with her family.

Wendy had always thought of menopause as a natural process, and she expected to go through it, in a word, naturally. But there was nothing natural-seeming about feeling tired, grouchy, sweaty, and hungry all at once. She felt she would go to any lengths to correct her feelings, even if it meant going on the estrogen supplements she had previously held in contempt.

In most doctors' offices, Wendy would have been diagnosed as menopausal and started on the usual cookbook recipe for menopause, a combination of pills with synthetic hormones. It wouldn't matter if she had arrived at menopause abruptly, following surgery, or slowly, following the usual course, or if she had bothersome symptoms or not. After all, to most doctors, menopause is menopause. But Wendy's best friend, whom we had once helped, asked her to see us for an evaluation.

After just a few minutes together, it was apparent to us that Wendy was suffering from a lifelong excess of estrogen. She had started making estrogen at a younger than average age; years of taking the older form of birth control pills followed by four years of hormone treatments only added to the amount of estrogen in her system.

Even more, because she was unable to become pregnant, Wendy had continued to ovulate and make yet more estrogen, rather than carrying and nursing a baby, which reduces the body's estrogen levels.

Her body also showed visible signs of estrogen excess. She had a fibroid (a benign, estrogen-sensitive tumor) in the uterus. Her bone density was 130 percent of the expected density for a woman her size and age, also a result of too much estrogen. (Since estrogen builds bone, the more estrogen, the denser the bones. This is why women with very dense bones have much higher rates of breast cancer—more estrogen promotes more breast cancer.)

And, the estrogen level in her blood was 350, or more than three times the usual amount for someone who's fifty.

It was clear that the objective here was not to supplement estrogen, but rather to block the high levels of estrogen—not only to help alleviate Wendy's symptoms, but also to reduce her risk of breast cancer from so much estrogen exposure.

We started Wendy on a program of exercise to reduce estrogen levels. We increased her fiber intake to speed elimination of estrogen from the gut as well as upping her intake of estrogen-balancing foods such as soy, flaxseed, and whole grains. She also started on supplements of black cohosh, vitamin E, and whole soy tablets containing genistein, and she reduced her alcohol and caffeine intake.

Six weeks later all of her symptoms were either gone or substantially improved. She felt good, was losing some weight, and was sleeping better. The lesson: Menopause wasn't making her sick. And if she had started on the standard treatment, she would only have increased her estrogen exposure, and probably her risk of breast cancer—not to mention blood clots, gallstones, hypertension, and weight gain.

In summary: Just because you have been diagnosed with a disease doesn't mean that you know your problem, or what's going to happen, or even how best to deal with it. The conditions that affect most people in this country are not necessarily diagnosable diseases. They are the result of a series of events, a domino effect that begins with the five forces of illness discussed in Part II. Simply naming the disease doesn't explain how or why you came down with the symptoms. And unless the how and why are addressed, the treatment just covers up the symptoms, or addresses only one aspect of the illness. Quite simply, this approach will never lead to true health.

## SUBMYTH: MENOPAUSE IS A DISEASE OF ESTROGEN DEFICIENCY

This one is just outright wrong.

Traditionally, women's symptoms related to menopause, such as hot flashes, night sweats, and sleep disturbance, are diagnosed as the disease called estrogen deficiency. The treatment is estrogen "replacement" therapy.

But we say that menopausal symptoms are not a disease—nor are they caused by estrogen deficiency. We believe that the widespread acceptance of this myth has created tremendous harm, because it has unnecessarily increased women's risk for cancer, heart disease, and stroke, and often exacerbated their uncomfortable symptoms as well.

The truth is that during the time leading up to menopause (or *perimenopause*), when symptoms are the most bothersome, estrogen levels are actually higher and more erratic than average.

The myth of menopause as estrogen deficiency is one of the most widely accepted in the area of women's health, and has been largely advanced by the pharmaceutical industry. The drug Premarin accounts for 70 percent of the world's prescriptions for estrogen, and is the fifth most commonly taken medication overall after acetaminophen (the active ingredient in the medication Tylenol and many other over-the-counter analgesics), ibuprofen, aspirin, and pseudoephedrine.

Premarin is the oldest of all of the forms of estrogen replacement, and it remains the most popular. This is surprising, considering it's made not of human but of horse estrogen. The name tells the story: Pre-mar-in is a blend of horse estrogens, made from pregnant mares' urine. We don't know of any reason why women should still be taking a horse's estrogen when their own natural estrogen has been available for over fifteen years in the form of Estradiol.

(Even more frightening is the fact that after the pregnant mare's foals are born, the drug company ships some of them off to be slaughtered, so the terrified babies' lives consist of being snatched from their mothers, thrown into the back of a truck, then tossed off the truck and butchered.)

The truth is that estrogen levels do not actually decline until a woman has stopped menstruating altogether, and even then most women are still producing some estrogen. The widespread cookbook therapy of giving all women estrogen to treat menopause has led to many serious complications, including breast and uterine cancer, blood clots, gallstones, high blood pressure, growth of uterine fibroids or fibrocystic breasts, migraines, weight gain, and even strokes and heart attacks. These are all known and well-described complications of Premarin, and are listed in every doctor's standard dictionary of drug therapy, the *Physicians' Desk Reference,* or *PDR.* Even worse, Premarin has been on the government's National Toxicology Program list of known carcinogens for over five years.

To make matters still worse, the primary reason doctors say they prescribe Premarin is to prevent heart attack and stroke in menopausal women. Large, controlled studies reporting their results over the past two years have now completely debunked this myth—the best studies available actually show that women prescribed Premarin had higher rates of heart attack than women not given estrogen at all.

It's hard to estimate how many thousands of women have been adversely affected by the widespread acceptance of these menopause myths, but in 2001 there were 46 million prescriptions written for Premarin. Finally, after years of recommendations to the contrary, the American Heart Association issued a position paper to physicians in July 2001 calling for the official debunking of the belief that Premarin is good for the heart.

Let's now look at Elaine, a forty-nine-year-old artist who had begun experiencing hot flashes, sleeping problems, and what she described as "brain fog"—she often felt tired and confused.

Her menstrual cycles were heavier than usual, and the PMS symptoms that used to last a few days were now lasting two weeks or more.

Elaine had been fit, active, and healthy; she ate well and hadn't been taking any medications until her doctor suggested Premarin to treat her symptoms and "to protect her heart from menopause."

After starting on Premarin, Elaine found her appetite increased—she experienced an insatiable desire for sweets, especially chocolate. She quickly gained fifteen pounds, most of it in her stomach, and she was horrified to see that she had developed a potbelly.

When she questioned her doctor, she again convinced Elaine to continue on the Premarin because of the protection it afforded. Elaine did feel her hot flashes had diminished somewhat, and she was sleeping a bit better, so she decided to continue.

Next, Elaine began experiencing headaches. A nurse suggested that she check her blood pressure. It was 160/90—Elaine had never had a reading that high before.

She soon returned to her doctor, who also found a high blood pressure reading and started Elaine on a diuretic medication to bring it down. The doctor attributed the new high blood pressure to Elaine's weight gain and suggested she go on a diet.

Things took a turn for the worse. Elaine's blood work came back with high cholesterol and high triglyceride levels (which may indicate possible heart disease, brain deterioration, and, potentially, stroke).

The triglycerides, her doctor said, had risen due to the sugar. She didn't tell Elaine that the Premarin might be causing both the rise in blood pressure and the rise in triglycerides, as well as the weight gain.

The problem was that Elaine now had too much estrogen. When we saw her, we found that she indeed also had high triglycerides, as well as evidence of inflammation. And she had elevated levels of the important clotting factor fibrinogen in her bloodstream, putting her at risk for blood clots and heart attack.

Again, our solution was simple. We stopped the Premarin and recommended lifestyle changes (including more exercise and a better, caffeine- and sugar-free diet), supplements including vitamin E and vitamin B complex, and such herbal remedies as Dong Quai and black cohosh. We also put her on a very low, temporary dose of estrogen (the new FDA-approved human [or bio-identical] estrogen, synthesized from soybeans as opposed to a horse's estrogen), transmitted through the skin in the form of a patch.

This very low dose of estrogen was sufficient to eliminate Elaine's symptoms, but did not have the negative side effects of Premarin. In three months, Elaine lost ten pounds; her levels of cholesterol, triglycerides, C-reactive protein (an indicator of inflammation in the bloodstream, which is one of the prime risk factors for heart attack and stroke), and fibrinogen were back to normal; and her blood pressure had also decreased. Eventually we were able to reduce and then eliminate the estrogen patch altogether.

### SUBMYTH: DEPRESSION CAUSES DEPRESSION

This one might sound silly, yet when you ask most doctors about depression, the argument can get senselessly circular. "Why am I depressed?" you ask. "Because you've come down with depression," the doctor says. "What are its symptoms?" you ask. "Loss of appetite, maybe some weight gain, sleeplessness, and worst of all, depression."

We don't think that depression causes depression. We feel that depression is caused by many factors, some psychological, some physiological, some genetic, and some that may not fall into any of these categories.

Because we don't believe this submyth, treating depression has become one of the more successful areas of our practice. Our method of identifying and targeting depression's root causes produces better results than those of most doctors who use a standard trial-and-error method backed by a battery of often futile medications.

The point is that the origin of depression may be physical, such as deficiency of omega-3 fatty acids, folate, or $B_{12}$, rather than mental. As another example, the bacteria in your gut can affect your brain chemistry; these bacteria release substances that can cause depression because they interfere with the brain's neurotransmitters (the chemicals in our brain that are involved with mood and thinking).

One of our patients, Hannah, had precisely this problem. Having had a history of depression, Hannah had tried the usual list of antidepressants, but each just seemed to work for only a few weeks before becoming ineffective.

When we talked with her, however, she also mentioned that she was experiencing severe digestive problems, including bloating and gas. Acting on this clue, we took a urine test, which showed an elevated level of DHPPA, a derivative of a common amino acid found in food. The bacteria in the gut alters the amino acid phenylalanine, and turns it into a chemical called DHPPA. This DHPPA was now effecting Hannah's brain chemistry by interfering with her neurotransmitters; this, in turn, was creating her depression.

For treatment, we prescribed Flagyl, an antibiotic that kills these bacteria (we also made sure she took probiotics so that the drugs didn't deplete all the health-promoting bacteria in Hannah's system).

Two weeks later, Hannah called to say that she felt as though she'd been living in the dark for years, and now she could finally see the light again. We recommended that Hannah continue to follow up with her psychiatrist, but we also put her on a maintenance program to promote a normal intestinal ecology.

In a nice turn of events, Mark Hyman recently taught a continuing-education course for doctors on our new paradigm of medicine; in the audience was a women who asked question after question. Finally he asked her why she was so curious. It turned out that she had been Hannah's psychiatrist for ten years and had had such little success with her that she was dying to know what had alleviated Hannah's depression.

### SUBMYTH: HEART DISEASE IS A DISEASE OF THE HEART

We don't believe that all heart disease is necessarily a problem with the heart itself. More important is circulation, or the arteries that supply the heart with oxygen and fuel from the blood. When these pipes are clogged, heart damage results. The heart itself is just an innocent bystander.

Most likely, the same process that clogs the pipes leading to and from the heart is simultaneously clogging all the other pipes—the ones that go to the brain, to the arms and legs, to the kidneys, and so on. So performing bypass surgery on the heart is simply a makeshift remedy—the patient is simply getting new pipes, which will soon be clogged again. And all the pipes going to the brain, the limbs, the kidneys are still just as clogged, because a heart bypass doesn't fix any of those other arteries.

Those doctors who are interested in the pipes leading to the heart think they know the culprit: cholesterol. But they're wrong. Cholesterol isn't always bad. Long-term studies (published in *The Lancet*, vol. 358, 2001) of octogenarians have actually shown that the higher the cholesterol, the lower the risk of death from all causes!

In fact, the octogenarians with the lowest cholesterol levels (less than 140) had the highest risk of death. Of course this only applies if you're eighty years old; it doesn't apply if you're forty or fifty. The reason? If you've lived to eighty years and have high cholesterol, then it must not be the dangerous kind of high cholesterol. Why? Because cardiovascular disease is really a disease of inflammation:

Only high cholesterol combined with inflammation seems to cause blockages in the pathways that lead to the heart.

Inflammation is the activation of your immune system. When the immune system is turned on, it's as though your body's defenses have entered search-and-destroy mode, as the aggressive white blood cells course through your bloodstream looking for an enemy to attack.

Among the victims caught in the crossfire of these fighting white blood cells are the arteries themselves. In the process of activating the immune system, the lining of the arteries becomes damaged, and wherever this damage occurs, cholesterol begins to accumulate in that artery.

Thus the inflammation designed to battle a problem causes a problem. Without inflammation, cholesterol does not appear to accumulate. A recent article in the *Journal of the American Medical Association* (July 4, 2001) corroborated this conclusion, as did a piece in the *New England Journal of Medicine* (June 17, 1999): Patients with inflammation, even those with low cholesterol, could prevent heart attack by taking statins (anticholesterol drugs) to reduce inflammation.

(What causes inflammation? You will read more about inflammation in Part II, but infections, stress, sugar, trans fats, toxins, lack of exercise, and malnutrition are all sources of inflammation. Allergies can also cause it, as can obesity and insulin resistance.)

Yet when faced with heart disease, doctors recommend a bypass. By so doing, we think, they bypass the real problem. Bypasses are the single most commonly performed unnecessary surgery in the country. Only two groups have been shown to benefit from bypass surgery: one, those whose arteries are so badly clogged that the heart can no longer beat adequately, and two, those with severe blockage in the main artery to the heart and signs of resulting poor blood flow.

# MYTH 3: DRUGS CURE DISEASE

Both of us still see children now and then (and Mark Liponis's wife is a pediatrician), so we try to keep on top of current events in pediatrics. The story we hear most often concerns children's ear infections.

Take the case of a young boy named Matthew, whose doctor had put him on the antibiotic amoxicillin, the accepted treatment for such infections. The drugs seemed to work—but not for long. Four weeks later the ear infection took a turn for the worse and Matthew returned to his doctor, who, thinking that Matthew needed a stronger antibiotic, prescribed Ceclor, which did the trick—for a while. Six weeks later, Matthew's infection worsened, so the doctor tried a still stronger antibiotic.

Antibiotics weren't what was needed. In fact, the infection was becoming more and more powerful because Matthew's well-meaning doctor was aggravating the situation. The increasingly stronger antibiotics were making it more and more difficult for the infection to improve.

Why? It's not just that antibiotics don't always cure infections. They can actually worsen them. When taken frequently, they may trigger mutations in bacteria, making those bacteria resistant. Stronger and stronger antibiotics are then necessary to kill these bacteria—perhaps until none is left that works.

The solution to Matthew's problem had nothing to do with drugs. It turned out the boy had an allergic reaction to milk, which was congesting his ears and creating the infection. So we took him off milk. Presto! The infection disappeared. Recent studies have confirmed that there is no difference in outcome for children treated with antibiotics compared with those who weren't treated at all.

Another example: Norman, a young stockbroker, came to us complaining of heartburn. Norman's doctor had told him to take the most powerful among the over-the-counter antacids, which Norman did, and as stronger and stronger pills appeared on the market, he continued to follow his doctor's orders, always taking the most potent.

These antacids are indeed effective in shutting down acid production in the stomach. The problem arises when patients who have been taking these pills for a prolonged period eventually stop taking them, creating a rebound effect that raises acid levels even higher than before. The symptoms intensify, and the patient then starts taking twice as many antacids to get relief. (The rebound effect is the result of acid-producing cells overcompensating for the previous blocking action of the drug; although this process is well known, it is not precisely understood.)

The culprit for excess acid reflux often isn't stomach acid, anyway, but a problem with the muscular sphincter that keeps the stomach contents inside the stomach. Heartburn sufferers usually have a poor diet; they tend to eat large meals as well as ingest too much alcohol, caffeine, and saturated fats. Thus, taking antacids isn't the answer. Diet is.

Heartburn sufferers may suffer from inadequate levels of magnesium (which relaxes the sphincter), or of hydrochloric acid, which is needed to activate the digestive forces, or even an infection with *H. pylori,* a newly discovered bacterium that can lead to indigestion, ulcers, and even stomach cancer. They may have diabetes, or be taking a medication that overrelaxes the muscular sphincter at the bottom of the esophagus. The symptoms are the same, but the cause may be different from individual to individual. The body has only so many ways of saying ouch.

★  ★  ★

Whatever the ailment, the problem is that conventional medicine uses drugs to interfere with, rather than to support, human biology. In other words, drugs end up blocking, or stopping, natural bio-chemical and/or physiologic processes. We take an antacid to block acid, an antianxiety pill to block certain stress-producing chemicals in the brain, an antibiotic to kill bacteria.

This isn't right. Think about it. When the smoke alarm goes off, you don't go upstairs and unplug it to stop the beeping. But that's what most prescription drugs usually do—they stop the alarm. They cover up symptoms, but they don't help you find out where the fire is.

Of course, drugs can be extremely helpful in many situations, par-ticularly in the short run. If you wake up with a headache one morning, try an aspirin. It usually works. But if you suffer from a chronic headache, aspirin may not be the best solution. It might even make your headache worse by giving you an analgesic rebound headache (if you've been taking acetaminophen or aspirin on a regular basis, stopping its use can actually cause your headache to intensify).

Likewise, if you have joint pain and take nonsteroidal anti-inflammatory drugs such as ibuprofen, your pain may decrease, but the joint destruction continues. These drugs may actually lead to accelerated joint damage, which can progress to the point where you may need joint replacement surgery—because people who take these painkillers, and who thereby feel less pain, are more apt to engage in activities that damage their joints. (Interesting new research also suggests that these drugs may worsen joint inflamma-tion and deterioration by interfering with the circulation to the joints themselves.)

In fact, most drugs are designed to interfere with the body's nat-ural functioning, due to conventional medicine's acute care model: Something hurts right now, let's fix it right now. Applying this acute care model to the management of chronic or long-term conditions, however, does not always produce a beneficial long-term result.

For example, a common class of diabetes medications, sulfonylureas, are often prescribed for people with Type 2 diabetes (the adult-onset form of the disease). These medications lower blood sugar by raising your insulin production. In the short term, raising your insulin will indeed lower your blood sugar. However, over time, these drugs stop working, because your body gets used to that higher insulin level. The higher your level of insulin in the long run, the more resistant to the insulin you become. (These drugs have actually been shown to *increase* heart disease, the main cause of death in diabetics.)

Although anti-inflammatory and diabetes medications may seem to be working for a while, they are actually worsening your condition. Eventually, your doctor may give up and prescribe insulin shots in massive and escalating doses just to keep your blood sugar under control—leading to an ever-worsening cycle of weight gain, high blood pressure, and high cholesterol, all direct results of insulin therapy.

Doctors rarely address the reasons someone has developed diabetes in the first place, although they have historically thought that adult-onset diabetes is caused by too little insulin. That's wrong. The problem is actually too much insulin, and increasing resistance to the insulin you normally produce. Conventional medicine shoots at the wrong target; adult-onset diabetes is caused by failure of the body to respond properly to insulin.

To deal properly with this condition, our goal is to lower the output of insulin and restore the body's sensitivity to the insulin it makes naturally. The key is to avoid drugs, and instead change your diet, control your weight, and exercise regularly. This means cutting out sugar, as well as anything the body converts to sugar quickly, such as refined grains, processed carbohydrates, and starches. It's also important to change your pattern of eating from two or three large meals a day to smaller, more frequent meals. Exercise and certain targeted supplements are also very important.

This approach to diabetes will lead to the elimination, rather than the escalation, of medications.

The list of drugs with harmful consequences is extensive: Anti-inflammatory drugs used to treat arthritis have been shown to increase the progression of the disease (and long-term use of anti-inflammatories such as cortisone often leads to diabetes, obesity, cataracts, stomach ulcers, high blood pressure, and osteoporosis); overdosing from acetaminophen is the leading cause of liver failure in Great Britain; drugs for Parkinson's disease often make its symptoms much worse.

According to the June 1999 issue of the *New England Journal of Medicine,* anti-inflammatory drugs account for more than 16,000 deaths a year due to intestinal hemorrhaging: "If deaths from gastrointestinal toxic effects from NSAIDs [nonsteroidal anti-inflammation drugs] were tabulated separately in the National Vital Statistics reports, these effects would constitute the fifteenth most common cause of death in the United States. Yet these toxic effects remain mainly a silent epidemic, with many physicians and most patients unaware of the magnitude of the problem. Furthermore the mortality statistics do not include deaths ascribed to the use of over-the-counter NSAIDS."

Not only are these statistics considered conservative, the figures cited include only prescription NSAIDs used to treat only arthritis and only in the United States. If prescription and over-the-counter NSAID-related hospitalizations and death rates were counted for all conditions, and throughout the world, the death count would be enormous.

In 2001, according to the National Institute for Healthcare Management Research and Educational Foundation, all of the top five best-selling drugs were designed to treat conditions that we feel can be dealt with in healthier ways. These drugs go by the brand names Lipitor, Prilosec, Prevacid, Zocor, and Celebrex (two are for heartburn, two are for high cholesterol, and one is for inflammation).

Prilosec and Prevacid, for example, are used to treat reflux and heartburn. Reflux (or gastroesophageal reflux) is the process that occurs when stomach contents, usually a combination of stomach acid and food, splash back up into the esophagus (the swallowing pipe that connects your mouth with your stomach). The stomach has a lining that protects it from the corrosive effects of stomach acid, but the esophagus lacks this protective lining. So when stomach acid splashes back up into it, the esophagus is burned, creating the sensation of heartburn.

The anti-heartburn drugs work by neutralizing the acid in the stomach, so if the contents of the stomach do back up into the esophagus, they won't produce a burning sensation. However, the truth is we're supposed to have acid in the stomach. Acid is critical to digesting food and absorbing nutrients. Calcium is a good example—it's not absorbed unless there's enough acid in the stomach. Acid is also present to kill the germs we ingest. Otherwise, they would go happily through our gastrointestinal tract. And stomach acid is critical for preventing bacteria from growing, as well as for activating certain digestive enzymes, which are stimulated only under certain acidic conditions.

Furthermore, without stomach acid, bacteria and yeast will start to grow in the small intestine, leading to irritable bowel syndrome and poor digestion, which, in turn, lead to more problems, such as abdominal pain, diarrhea, and nausea.

Instead of too much stomach acid, the source of the problem lies with the sphincter that separates the stomach from the esophagus. There are actually three sphincters: the lower esophageal sphincter, which separates the esophagus from the stomach; the pyloric sphincter, which separates the stomach from the small intestine; and the anal sphincter. The second one sits at the outlet of the stomach, the pylorus. This sphincter must be stimulated by the parasympathetic nervous system (the part of our nervous system that causes relaxation) to open and let food out of the stomach and into the small intestine.

In order for your digestive juices to flow properly, or in order for them to flow in the right direction (namely, south), you need to have all the sphincters working correctly, opening so the food can leave your stomach.

However, these three sphincters can malfunction for a number of reasons, including stress, infections, and nutrient deficiencies. (For example, a magnesium deficiency will lead to general problems with all three sphincters and can cause tight, spastic muscles all over the body. Constipation is a classic example of a problem caused by magnesium deficiency—which is why one of the classic treatments for constipation is milk of magnesia, or a big dose of magnesium. But if you take acid blockers, the drugs will prevent you from absorbing the needed magnesium, creating a vicious cycle.)

Overeating can also be a cause of heartburn and indigestion, as it puts more pressure on the lower esophageal sphincter, as can food sensitivities or allergies, or a bad diet. Several substances, including alcohol, chocolate, caffeine, and fats, can cause the lower esophageal sphincter to relax and cause reflux.

Drugs also effect these sphincters. The worst offenders are calcium channel blockers used to treat high blood pressure; steroids, such as Prednisone (used for arthritis, lupus, and inflammatory conditions); and statins (cholesterol-lowering drugs).

To treat a problem, you must remove the cause. If symptoms persist, then stress reduction, a change in diet, or perhaps herbal therapy may help. Drugs are not usually necessary.

Yet the drug companies want to convince you otherwise. They benefited from the disease now known as GERD (gastroesophageal reflux disease) because, when it was discovered that antibiotics cured ulcers, there was no longer a market for their high-priced antacid medications. (A recent study compared the efficacy of an antibiotic and high-powered expensive antacids in treating ulcers; the antibiotic turned out to be just as effective and far less expensive.)

So the drug companies found a new use for their preexisting drugs with the designation of GERD, which used to have the simple name heartburn, and which most people treated inexpensively with antacids. But now that GERD is a full-fledged disease, the drug companies want you to fight it with high-priced prescription acid blockers.

In 2001 spending on prescription drugs shot up 18.8 percent, to $131.9 billion, according to a study by the National Institute for Health Care Management Foundation, a nonprofit, nonpartisan group that conducts research on health care issues.

Alan F. Holmer, president of the Pharmaceutical Research and Manufacturers of America, the main trade association for drug companies, responded, "This report should be hailed as good news" because it means that "more patients are getting more and better medicines."

But we couldn't disagree more. Good news? That more and more people are spending more and more of their money on drugs they don't need? In 2001, 2.8 billion prescriptions were filled in the United States, or an average of 9.9 per person. We think that drug industry prescriptions have gotten far out of hand. Doctors have been bribed and brainwashed by pharmaceutical companies to prescribe new, expensive medications for every ailment—even when a simple change in lifestyle or diet can accomplish the same or a better result. Salesmen never come to a doctor's office to explain how patients could reduce their heartburn by cutting back on coffee, alcohol, fat, or chocolate, or by taking magnesium.

As with the case of GERD, the drug companies benefit from the designation of new diseases to fit their current supply of drugs, and then market them as such. For example, Prozac: Once marketed for depression, drugmaker Eli Lilly recently targeted a new disease Prozac can cure. Television commercials now ask women if they have the "disease" coined premenstrual dysphoric disorder, or PDD. Up until recently PDD was simply PMS (premenstrual syndrome), but women would not have bought Prozac to treat that, so the company relabeled the symptoms and announced that they require a prescription medication to cure. And rather than simply selling it as rebottled Prozac, the company has reissued it with the catchy name Sarafem.

Do these companies really have your interests in mind? Johnson & Johnson had to remove Zomax, a highly successful anti-inflammatory drug, from the market after it caused fourteen deaths from severe allergic reactions. Eli Lilly's drug Oraflex, another anti-arthritis drug, was also pulled after seventy deaths occurred after its release. Weight loss drugs such as Redux and the combination known as Fen-Phen were also pulled when they appeared to be causing lung and heart-valve damage. The cardiac drug Enkaid was removed from the market when it caused dangerous and lethal heart arrhythmias and thousands of deaths. The antihistamine Seldane was taken off the shelves after it was found to cause potentially lethal heart irregularities when taken in combination with other common medications. DES was given to thousands of women in the 1950s to ward off miscarriages—until it was discovered that not only was it ineffective, it caused breast cancer in some women, as well as vaginal cancer, birth defects, and infertility in their daughters.

Even though such drugs are tested on animals and several hundred people before the FDA (the U.S. Food and Drug Administration) clears them for public use, the real experiments don't start until millions of people start taking them.

We think it doesn't make sense to try any of these new drugs until they've stood the test of time after their release into the marketplace, unless, of course, they represent a breakthrough category that offers a benefit unmatched by any already proven drug.

We also believe that there are better ways to treat symptoms that don't involve drugs. This is what we told Rudy, a fifty-four-year-old fireman who had worked his way up to captain before a chronic back problem put him on permanent disability. Rudy had first noticed back problems in his thirties, when a few Tylenol a day were enough to keep him on the job. Over the years, however, his pain increased and he finally consulted his doctor, who diagnosed Rudy with arthritis in his spine and began giving him prescription anti-inflammatory drugs and pain medication.

Each new medicine would work for a few months, or even up to a year, but then the effect would wear off and Rudy would be immobilized with pain again. This process escalated as he took stronger and stronger medications.

Three years ago Rudy was overcome by an ominous wave of weakness and he passed out. His crew rushed him to a hospital, where he began passing large amounts of blood rectally; he was immediately given two blood transfusions and admitted to the intensive care unit, where the cause of his attack was determined: Rudy had a large ulcer in his stomach caused by the arthritis medicines he was taking for his back.

His condition stabilized, Rudy spent a week in the hospital and took medications for another six weeks to heal the ulcer. But in the meantime, he could no longer take the arthritis anti-inflammatory medications. So the back pain grew, and his doctor responded by prescribing narcotic medications such as codeine.

Rudy soon became addicted to these stronger painkillers; his job performance also suffered as the narcotics made him feel foggy.

Rudy asked if there were any alternatives, so his doctor ordered an MRI scan of Rudy's back to see if surgery might help the problem. The scan showed considerable arthritis in the lower spine and areas where the nerves were being pinched by newly developed bone spurs; the doctor announced that Rudy had a condition known as spinal stenosis and referred him to a neurosurgeon for possible surgery. After looking at the scan, the neurosurgeon told Rudy that surgery might help, but there was no guarantee that it would relieve his pain—and there was a small chance of paralysis from the surgery itself.

"Aren't there any other options?" Rudy asked. The neurosurgeon recommended Rudy see a pain specialist for a cortisone injection in his back. Although he was leery of taking cortisone, Rudy saw it as his only option. He took the cortisone shots and the pain specialist put him on a low dose of an oral cortisone called prednisone.

It felt like magic. For the first time in over twenty years, Rudy had no pain in his back at all. But like the other treatments, this didn't last—within six months the pain returned. So his doctor increased the dosage of prednisone, which helped a little, but now Rudy noticed that he was gaining weight—within four months he had gained eighteen pounds, and almost all of it was right around the middle of his body.

Even more alarming, Rudy's blood pressure had risen. Rudy's doctor prescribed blood pressure medication, too. And because Rudy's cholesterol level had increased by eighty points, he started Rudy on Zocor to lower it.

Rudy, feeling like a walking pharmacy, decided enough was enough and scheduled the back surgery, which, according to his neurosurgeon, was successful.

But to Rudy's surprise, while he was in the hospital he was diagnosed with diabetes and had to take insulin shots to keep his blood sugar under control. His doctor explained that the steroids had caused him to become diabetic. And since he had been on prednisone for so long prior to his hospital visit, his doctors now gave him doses of intravenous steroids during his surgery, which made his blood sugar rise even higher.

Thankfully, his back pain was more bearable, although not completely gone. But Rudy paid a high price for this relief. He was now taking medications for diabetes, high blood pressure, high cholesterol, and ulcers, not to mention a small dose of steroids; moreover, his doctor had put him on Prozac when he was discharged from the hospital.

Rudy wondered if he had made the right decision about having surgery—he was no longer able to work and was placed on complete disability, making him feel even worse. After all, he'd always been a fireman, and he was only fifty-four years old. Rudy was feeling both hopeless and helpless about his situation until he arrived at Canyon Ranch.

Rudy's history told us most of the story, and a few blood and urine tests confirmed what we suspected as we backtracked the path of Rudy's problems and re-created a dangerous but common chain of events.

Rudy's back problem was never properly taken care of when he was thirty. Rather than taking medications to cover up the symptoms, Rudy should have been on a restorative program of stretching and strengthening to prevent his back from getting worse. Instead, all those medications led to further problems: The arthritis pills gave him a bleeding ulcer; the steroids caused weight gain, diabetes, and high cholesterol; and the downward spiral led to depression.

But there was hope. These problems were neither permanent nor irreversible. All of Rudy's problems could be corrected with changes in diet, lifestyle, and exercise.

First, we put Rudy on a low-glycemic diet. We asked him to reduce or eliminate any sources of sugar, or anything his body would convert to sugar, such as refined grains, processed carbohydrates, and starches. By doing this (and with the help of a nutritional supplement program), we were able to get his cholesterol level in check. We also started him on an exercise program; he found he was able to get a great workout with water aerobics, and he really began to enjoy it when he found it didn't bother his back at all—in fact, he felt better. Rudy also took a few treatments of directed massage, or neuromuscular therapy, and some additional physical therapy as well.

Rudy started feeling better and better. He found he was losing weight for the first time in several years, and he didn't even feel like he was dieting. In fact, his appetite, which was voracious while taking the prednisone, was hardly noticeable. When Rudy left Canyon Ranch we gave him a program to follow at home that helped him taper off his medications, and we scheduled him for some follow-up blood work in six weeks.

When we talked to Rudy again, he had already lost twelve pounds. His back no longer hurt, and in addition to working out in the pool, he was now able to go to the gym and use the elliptical machine and some light hand weights. He had quit Prozac; he didn't think he needed it. His cholesterol had dropped ninety points, his blood sugar was now normal, and there was substantially less inflammation in his bloodstream. Rudy's blood pressure was in the normal range at 120/70 every day, his heartburn was gone, and he was able to cut his ulcer medication in half.

Eight weeks later Rudy was still making steady progress. He was also proud to announce that he had been back to his local doctor, who, astounded, stopped all of Rudy's medications. Rudy was now twenty-six pounds lighter than when he had arrived at Canyon Ranch. And he felt great!

★　　★　　★

Rudy's story is not uncommon. Every week we see people suffering from clear, curable, and unnecessary symptoms that are directly caused by medications prescribed in the right dose for the right reason by a well-meaning doctor. But when symptoms occur, doctors are more likely to diagnose a condition and prescribe a new medication than to examine the possibility that the new symptom was caused by one or more of their medications.

Just last month we received a panicked phone call from June, whom we had seen several months previously for help with menopausal symptoms. She was horrified because her doctor was referring her to a hematologist/oncologist to rule out possible bone marrow cancer.

When we asked her to tell us the details, she said that due to severe bladder infections she had seen two urologists, and each had prescribed antibiotics to treat the infection. Over the past six weeks she had been on three different antibiotics.

Because she was wondering what might be causing three urinary tract infections back-to-back, June consulted her internist, who checked her blood counts. June told us that her blood showed a very low white blood cell count (the cells that fight infection). Her doctor thought that she was getting infections because of this low level of white blood cells, and that they may have been low as a result of cancer of the bone marrow, so she referred June to a hematologist/oncologist. Needless to say, June was terrified.

It took all of sixty seconds to pinpoint the problem. The medication June was taking, Macrodantin, can affect the bone marrow and lower the white blood cell count. We explained the problem and told June to stop taking the antibiotic and repeat her blood count in three weeks.

June called us three weeks later to report that her blood counts were normal again and to say thanks.

★    ★    ★

The increasingly popular cholesterol drugs raise these same issues. When you take a drug to lower your cholesterol, it doesn't change the insulin resistance that raised your cholesterol in the first place, it doesn't change your blood sugar problem, it doesn't lower your blood pressure or your homocysteine level or the amount of iron in the bloodstream—all of which are known risks that need to be addressed in order to reverse or control so-called heart disease. The cholesterol drug lowers cholesterol, making you think you are fine because your cholesterol is lower.

But the medication hasn't addressed the underlying reason why your cholesterol might be high to start with, as we told Albert, a three-hundred-pound patient who had recently suffered a heart attack. Albert was taking the standard heart attack treatment: Lipitor, beta-blocker, aspirin, and a low-fat diet.

But from a blood test we learned that Albert was severely insulin resistant. Even though the Lipitor was controlling his cholesterol, it was doing nothing for his insulin resistance. And despite the Lipitor, Albert continued to have high levels of triglycerides and dangerously low levels of the so-called good cholesterol, HDL (high-density lipoprotein). And he had sky-high insulin levels, as well as a substantial amount of inflammation in his bloodstream, as measured by his high C-reactive protein level.

As we said, the drugs simply weren't dealing with Albert's original problem, which was insulin resistance. So even though Albert thought he was doing well because his cholesterol was normal, he was still at high risk for a second heart attack because the underlying problem wasn't being addressed.

In fact, the other medications may have actually been aggravating the insulin resistance, since beta-blockers can worsen the biochemical and physiological aspects of insulin resistance. But because no one identified the insulin resistance, Albert wasn't placed on the appropriate therapy.

Luckily, we were able to straighten Albert out with a program targeted at improving insulin resistance; this included the proper diet, exercise, weight loss, and specific targeted supplements.

Doctors even fall for the myth that drugs cure disease when treating themselves. We recently met with a well-known midwestern physician who was taking many more drugs than most of his patients—one to get him to sleep, one to deal with his anxiety, one for depression, one to keep him awake, as well as one to help him work.

By the time he came to see us at Canyon Ranch, this poor man was thoroughly disoriented. It turned out he had a problem with vitamin $B_{12}$ deficiency, a known cause of cognitive dysfunction, dementia, and fatigue.

And consider the alarming increase in drug prescriptions for children. Mark Liponis's wife, a pediatrician, recently worked at a summer camp where a full 20 percent of the boys were medicated with psychotropic drugs. These were normal, middle-class kids from normal backgrounds taking Ritalin, Cylert, Prozac, Paxil, and/or Celexa or other drugs.

The problem is that for most practicing physicians, the prescription pad is their tool kit. Writing prescriptions is what they do. They don't have much else to offer someone. A doctor without a prescription pad is naked.

Recently we met a man who told his doctor that he was nervous because he was getting married and moving out of the country for a new job. His doctor immediately recommended a new antidepressant called Serzone. The man refused it, pointing out that you're supposed to be nervous when you get married, take a new job, and move to a new country. But doctors want to medicate you simply for living your life.

Rather than do that, we are attempting to help the body do what

it does normally, but do it better, which is why we have b
moting the use of what we call pro-drugs. Rather than fight
the natural processes of your body, a pro-drug works with
body to make it healthier.

After all, remedies don't have to be synthetic creations of the
pharmaceutical industry. Millions of arthritis sufferers have found
relief from their pain with nonprescription, natural supplements
called glucosamine and chondroitin sulfate. Glucosamine, a natural
substance present in the body, is also found in high quantities in the
shells of crustaceans such as crabs, lobster, and shrimp. Glucosamine
not only relieves symptoms, but reduces the joint damage that
occurs in arthritis; it puts out the fire as well as turning off the
smoke alarm.

Chondroitin is a member of a family of compounds called pro-
teoglycans, which combine protein and sugar molecules. Like glucosamine, chondroitin is found in the normal joint fluid, and it may
act as a lubricant of sorts. As a supplement, it is obtained from either
cow cartilage or from crustaceans' shells.

The glucosamine-chondroitin combination, one of our favorite
pro-drugs, works by improving the body's formation of cartilage,
and also by reducing inflammation of the joints themselves.

Another pro-drug is N-acetyl cysteine, or NAC, a naturally
occurring amino acid compound found in the body that augments
and improves the body's normal mechanisms that thwart illness and
disease.

NAC is used by many organs, particularly the liver; NAC helps it
produce antioxidants and detoxify. Our body always stores a certain
amount of NAC, but if those stores become depleted (when the
liver is overtaxed), the liver and other organs can be damaged.

NAC has been clinically proven to protect the liver from damage
that can occur from excess acetaminophen usage. Acetaminophen
requires NAC in the liver for its elimination. Excessive intake of

acetaminophen drains the NAC stores in the liver, and any further intake goes on to cause liver damage.

NAC has also been shown to protect the kidneys from damage when X-ray dye is administered for radiological imaging, as with CAT scans or angiograms. And according to an October 2001 study published in *Neurology*, Alzheimer's patients showed improvement in cognitive tasks after six months of treatment with NAC.

Still other examples of pro-drugs are alpha-lipoic acid and acetyl-L-carnitine. Like glucosamine and NAC, these compounds are widely available in most vitamin or natural food stores without a prescription. Alpha-lipoic acid (also known as thioctic acid) is another naturally occurring substance in the body; it is a potent antioxidant and anti-inflammatory. Research shows it can augment the body's healing mechanisms, as well as prevent and improve symptoms and disease for a wide range of conditions, including diabetes, neuropathy (nerve damage), liver disease, hypertension, hearing loss, and nerve damage in the brain associated with conditions such as Parkinson's disease.

Acetyl-L-carnitine (ALCAR), also a naturally occurring substance, has shown clinical benefits when used to treat a variety of conditions. Like alpha-lipoic acid, ALCAR has a protective effect on brain neurons and the liver.

These substances promote and improve normal patterns of cellular function and healing in many cells and organs. Ongoing clinical trials are studying the effects of these pro-drugs on a number of conditions, including degenerative diseases associated with aging.

We strongly favor the use of these pro-drugs whenever possible. Rather than combat the body's reaction to a particular stress, we prefer to augment and promote the body's natural healing mechanisms by (a) eliminating the source of the stress itself, and (b) using pro-drugs to enhance the body's normal protective and healing processes.

## SUBMYTH: IF THE FDA APPROVES A DRUG, IT IS SAFE

Not long ago one of our patients, a woman who works for the FDA, told us something we'd always suspected: While studies on any drug being reviewed, as well as the company's internal research, must be submitted to the FDA, not all of this information must be published for the public's perusal.

In other words, the drug companies practice full disclosure to the FDA, but not to the public. This means that negative data are seldom if ever seen outside the FDA. Moreover, some drugs don't even go through full testing. Many drugs are never tested at all among the elderly or the very young. Until recently, numerous drugs were never even tested on women—and the effects of most drugs on a developing fetus or pregnancy are still unknown. As of September 2001, just 22 percent of subjects were women in early drug trials. Only in 1994 did the NIH (National Institutes of Health) require analysis of outcomes of clinical trials according to the gender of the study subjects. Even now, 33 percent of new drug applications do not include separate safety and efficacy data for men and women, as required by the FDA.

Furthermore, most drugs are not tested for all the possible interactions that can occur when one drug is used in combination with others. Drugs are generally tested against other classes of drugs, rather than with each specific example of drugs within each class.

There's more: Popular drugs are often used in ways that differ from their original FDA-approved indication. For example, synthetic estrogen was never approved for its current use in lowering the risk of heart disease or the prevention of osteoporosis (in women). It was approved only for treating hot flashes. In fact, the *PDR* specifically states this drug should not be used to treat heart disease, as studies show it increases the risk of heart disease in women: "A recent four-year study suggests that women with a history of coronary heart disease may have an increased risk of serious cardiac events during the first year of treatment with estrogen/progestin therapy. Therefore, if you have had a heart attack, or you have been told you have blocked coronary arteries, or have any heart problem, you should consult your physician regarding the potential benefits and risks of estrogen/progestin therapy."

Many drugs, initially approved by the FDA, were later withdrawn because they were clearly dangerous. Rezulin was used by diabetics to control blood sugar. It was effective, but it also caused deaths from liver failure. Phenylpropanolamine (PPA) is a common decongestant that has been an ingredient in many over-the-counter sinus medications for years. It also has a mild stimulant and appetite-suppressant action, and for this reason has been an ingredient of over-the-counter weight-loss aids and diet pills, too. A study reported in the *New England Journal of Medicine* (April 5, 2001) found a fifteenfold increase in the risk of hemorrhagic stroke (bleeding inside the brain) in young, otherwise healthy women who had taken PPA in over-the-counter weight-loss products. The FDA has estimated that between two hundred and five hundred people suffer strokes every year as a result of PPA, which had been on the market for over fifty years, meaning it may have caused thousands of strokes during that time.

Why does this happen? One obvious reason: Everyone is different. When researchers study drugs, they look at their effects on the average white, 160-pound, thirty-year-old male. Yet not everyone is a white, 160-pound, thirty-year-old male. And people react differently to different drugs; certain ethnic groups, like African Americans or Asians, often have different reactions to blood pressure medications. But taking all this into account would cost too much.

Here's how the FDA works, in brief: Three phases of testing are required before a new drug can be approved. Phase I studies usually involve between twenty and eighty people (some animal studies are common prior to Phase I human trials). Phase II trials involve several hundred people. Phase III trials typically involve several hundred to several thousand people.

But if you start to divide even several thousand people by age, gender, race, and other characteristics such as concomitant medication usage, diet, weight, and alcohol or caffeine use, you end up with smaller and smaller numbers of study subjects in each group, making it much more difficult to compare these groups with control groups with similar characteristics. It also becomes prohibitively expensive to conduct trials in this manner. So more often than not, drugs are approved based on the study of more generalized and more available groups, such as young men.

We're not saying the FDA is a disaster by any means, because it does a remarkable amount of good work, on a tight budget, year after year after year. It's just that, like any other large organization, it's not anywhere near perfect.

So how do you best protect yourself?

Read those information sheets pharmacies must now distribute when they dispense a prescription. They explain what the drug is, how to take it, possible side effects, and more. And read the labels carefully—although you may scare yourself half to death. Just try a Tylenol label for a start.

We constantly see patients who say, "I feel achy," "I have diarrhea," "My skin is itchy," "My hair is falling out."

"What medications are you taking?" we ask. When we get the answer, we look for the side effects, and guess what they are? Achiness, diarrhea, itchiness, loss of hair. Yet people don't think that a drug their doctor prescribes for them could cause them to feel so bad.

Become aware of how you feel when you start on a medication. Many people take whatever their doctor prescribes. Soon they feel tired, swollen, constipated—whatever the side effects of the drug might be. These symptoms might suggest that this isn't the best medication for them. But people often shrug off the symptoms or think they have to put up with them. You don't. When you find the right medication for you, it won't have the same side effects.

There's good news in the not-too-far-off future. A new field called pharmacogenomics may eliminate this horrible process of being a human guinea pig; it uses genetic profiling to match an individual to an appropriate drug.

Let's say that you need to take a medication to lower your blood pressure. There are at least seven different classes of drugs on the market, including over sixty approved medications for high blood pressure. How does your doctor decide which to use? Normally this would be a process of trial and error. Wouldn't it be better if you could be tested beforehand to know exactly which drug is the most likely to be both effective and free of side effects?

Pharmacogenomics can offer that possibility. Here's how it works: Researchers take a drop of blood and put it on a special chip; the chip then profiles your genetic enzyme function as it relates to drug metabolism. These microchips can test your blood for the presence and activity of many of the thousands of specific enzymes in your liver that process and eliminate drugs. The chips can also test to see if you can handle a particular medication—drugs that may be toxic to one person aren't to another. And the chips may also be able to identify whether a particular person may require a higher level of a particular nutrient, vitamin, or mineral, in order to process certain medications efficiently.

Look for pharmacogenomics. And remember that drugs don't always cure disease. Sometimes, they can cause it.

# MYTH 4: YOUR GENES DETERMINE YOUR FATE

One of the most interesting stories from recent medical literature concerns the American Pima Indians. These people have lived in Arizona for centuries and were—until the 1950s—thin, fit, and healthy. Since then they have become the world's second-fattest population (the Samoans rank first). The Pimas have a staggeringly high 80 percent rate of diabetes. Their life expectancy is forty-six years.

The Pima Indians who live in Mexico, however, are thin and fit, with no incidence of diabetes at all. These people are genetically identical to their cousins across the border, but the state of their health couldn't be more different.

The Pimas in Mexico have lived the same healthy lifestyle as their ancestors. The Pimas in Arizona had fallen victim to what we call the White Menace (a diet replete with white flour, white sugar, and white fat—shortening, or trans fat). Their culture became over-consumptive, but undernourished, fat, and unhealthy. (It's quite possible to be both fat and malnourished, because if you're eating a great deal of food, but none of it is nutritious, that combination is a prescription for disease.)

The myth that genes are fixed and that they determine your health has been around for many decades. Conventional medicine's fascination with genetics has led doctors to forget an important truism: Genotypes differ from phenotypes. Your *genotype* is your inherent genetic blueprint. Your *phenotype* is your current physical being: the product of what you eat, how you take care of your body, and your state of mind.

Studies on twins have shown the same results: Identical twins (with the same genotype) who are raised in different environments can develop completely different phenotypes. Although these twins have identical genetic blueprints, they can end up looking quite different. One may be overweight and age poorly compared with the twin who is normal and aging well; such twins can also register different blood pressure and cholesterol levels—all subject to variations in their lifestyle, habits, diet, and so on. These people prove that you are not the predetermined and permanent product of your genes.

And yet, despite the preponderance of research on the subject, the myth of genetic determinism (that you are a prisoner of your parents' genes) continues to depress too many of our patients, causing them to believe they are doomed—or, in some cases, invulnerable, as we have also met several men and women who think they can afford to drink, smoke, and luxuriate in laziness because everyone in their family enjoys good health. (We tell them that yes, they can do these things—but they won't be able to do them for very long.)

Few people realize that our genes are not static, but dynamic— the active machinery of our biochemistry that operates day by day, moment by moment. Our genes represent the code, or template, from which proteins are made. All that genes do is store the information on this template. By storing the template for specific proteins, our genes can be passed on from cell to cell in the process of cell division, cell duplication, and reproduction.

Every cell in your body contains the same set of genes (with the exception of reproductive cells such as sperm or eggs [ova], and red blood cells, which lack a nucleus and hence lack DNA). So genes serve as a memory for the specific set of proteins required for any particular organism. In this context, the term *protein* refers to something much more complex than the simple concept of dietary protein. These proteins are incredibly diverse and complicated biological molecules and include thousands of enzymes, antibodies, structural proteins, messenger molecules, receptors, peptide hormones, cytokines, and many other compounds. Humans probably have somewhere around 30,000 genes—science has yet to figure out the exact number—but those genes code for more than 300,000 different proteins in each human being.

These proteins serve many functions, from providing the structure of our bodies to controlling the essential processes of energy production, and cellular and organ function.

Genes do provide a set of directions that help our body function, but it is a misconception that the *expression* of our genes cannot be changed. This may be true for the few traits that are controlled by a single gene. However, most of our physical and biochemical characteristics are controlled by many genes. Our height, our weight, our metabolism, our tendencies, and most illnesses, as well as our aging process, are affected by multiple genes in concert with our environment.

Many of these genes are also affected by nutrients, vitamins, and minerals that are involved in the chemical reactions within our cells.

The truth is, we all enjoy a tremendous opportunity to affect the expression of our genes—as well as our traits, tendencies, and overall health—by improving both our physical environment and our cellular environment via diet and lifestyle choices.

Here's one of the most unambiguous examples. Let's say you were born with a genetic tendency for heart disease. Meanwhile, you smoke, don't exercise, eat poorly, gain weight, and are under stress, which, taken together, strongly suggest you are likely to develop heart disease at an early age.

However, if you had that same genetic tendency for heart disease, but avoided smoking, exercised regularly, ate well, maintained your weight, reduced your stress, and maintained the proper intake of nutrients and antioxidants, you would quite likely prevent heart disease from ever developing.

Thus we can change our genes, or at least how they affect our health. By examining and correcting key imbalances, we can improve the outcome of our genetic inheritance and prevent many of the illnesses that were previously felt to be inevitable.

All of us carry genes that encode for a protein called APO E, or apolipoprotein E. This gene comes in several flavors—epsilon 2, epsilon 3, and epsilon 4. If you have APO E type 2, you're lucky. You possess what is nicknamed the "immortality gene," which means you may actually get away with smoking, eating poorly, and not exercising, and still live to be ninety. You are quite resistant to illness.

If you have epsilon 3 (like 80 percent of us), you must eat right, control your weight, exercise, and avoid bad habits to remain healthy.

A small percentage of the population have the epsilon 4 protein. Such individuals can eat right, exercise, and avoid smoking, but still may suffer from heart attacks, stroke, or Alzheimer's in their sixties and seventies.

Yet even those at the genetically worst end of the spectrum seem able to change the expression of that unfortunate gene. We recently met a woman who was ninety years old and still living independently; she even had a nine-to-five job as an accountant, and she engaged in many activities. Yet she carried the epsilon 4 gene. She managed to beat her bad luck by doing everything just right: diet, ultraprevention evaluations, supplements, and exercise. And new research shows that others with epsilon 4 can prevent disease with aggressive lifestyle choices and preventive therapies.

So yes, you can change your genetic inclination. Every cell has eighteen feet of DNA within it. Every person has 100 trillion cells. That's all information. Some of it is fixed. You cannot change your gender, race, or hair color (naturally, at least). But other genes are different.

Think about this: Most of your DNA is involved in maintaining your day-to-day biochemical functions, because everything your body does requires information from your DNA. Everything you do involves communication with your DNA, so basically you are talking to your genes every moment of your life. Whether you are eating, thinking, exercising, being exposed to toxins—it's all a form of communication with the outside world and your DNA. This concept of genes as learning, growing, and changing things is a new one, and is due to the revolution in molecular biology.

Each cell in our body has tens of thousands of different genes within it. The genes in every cell are an identical set, unique from person to person, but identical within each cell of a particular individual. Only a small fraction of these genes are being used in any cell at any particular point in time.

For example, our brain cells use a subset of these genes, our liver cells use a different subset of genes, and our muscle cells use yet another subset.

Which genes are selected for use depend on many factors, such as the cell type, the needs of the body or those particular cells, and the cellular processes that might be occurring, such as growth or repair, regeneration or reproduction. The way these genes are selected and expressed is also affected by the cellular environment, which in turn is affected by a person's nutrition, habits, lifestyle, energy, exposures, and the five forces of illness discussed in the next section (sludge, burnout, heat, waste, and rust).

That's how your phenotype (the expression of your genotype) is generated: The genes that are selected for use produce physical traits and characteristics that determine the visible and measurable appearance of the body—the thickness of the skin, the speed of the reflexes, the metabolic rate, the blood pressure, cholesterol level, and so on.

The point is that the process of gene selection, or *genetic expression,* can be directly affected by the environment in which the genes live. A bad environment often leads to poor genetic expression. If someone eats poorly, doesn't exercise, smokes, drinks excessively, or is under constant stress, it has a direct effect on the expression of the genes within his or her cells. We can therefore change and positively impact the genetic expression within our cells, leading to a healthier, more vital phenotype.

How did we travel down the wrong path for so long in thinking genes were unchangeable?

As mentioned, our understanding of genes originated with the work of Moravian monk Gregor Mendel, who determined that there are two genes for every trait, and that these genes are immutable. No one disputed this idea for more than a century.

But remember that Mendel had studied an extremely simple system: the pea plant. If you apply his logic to a human, how is it that in reality less than 1 percent of all the conditions that affect us are caused by mutation in a single gene—rare disorders at that, like cystic fibrosis and Tay-Sachs?

With these truly genetic diseases, the only hope for a cure lies in a technological solution, such as gene splicing or gene transfer. But because the mutation occurs in a gene that is always expressed, or "turned on," there is only so much that can be done to improve such conditions, even with an optimal cellular environment.

However, the vast majority of conditions that affect us are not caused by a defect in a single gene. They are the result of communication among many genes, and the various ways they interact with one another and their environment. That's why the expression of that group of genes depends on the individual and outside factors such as lifestyle and personal habits.

For example, there's a gene in the cells that line the colon that may determine whether or not you get colon cancer—it's a tumor-suppressor gene. This gene is turned on by a substance called butyrate, which is a type of fat produced by the healthy forms of bacteria that normally inhabit our colon, such as lactobacillus bacteria.

So by keeping the right bacteria in your gut and by eating enough fiber, you can turn on a gene that turns off cancer; the environment in the colon is that important, as it affects the genes that may prevent cancer.

Here's another example of illness that can be treated by influencing a gene: sickle-cell anemia, a disorder that can occur in African peoples when, under certain conditions of stress, the hemoglobin in red blood cells suddenly distorts, or "sickles" (normally round, the red blood cells turn sickle shaped, like a crescent moon).

These sickle-shaped cells, unable to pass smoothly through the body, become stuck in the capillaries of bones, joints, and organs, which leads to pain.

In looking for a solution to sickle-cell anemia, researchers found that they could change the genetic expression of DNA within the red blood cells. They discovered that the drug hydroxyurea can turn on dormant genes in the red blood cells that encode for the production of immature, or fetal, hemoglobin. Because fetal hemoglobin doesn't sickle like adult hemoglobin, sickle-cell patients given hydroxyurea are able to produce more of the fetal hemoglobin, which prevents their red blood cells from sickling. By altering the expression of genes within the red blood cells, many of the symptoms of sickle-cell anemia can be prevented.

Genes are very protected, and we can help keep them that way. Located at the center of each cell, genes are surrounded by a series of membranes and proteins called histones that ward off toxins, radiation, and mechanical harm. Without these defenses, our genes would be subject to damage and mutation leading to anything from cancer to birth defects.

These protective cell membranes and walls are composed largely of lipids, or fats, as well as carbohydrates and proteins. The types of fats, carbohydrates, and proteins that protect our genes are determined, in part, by our diet, so the food we eat literally helps create the environment in which our genes exist. If we put junk food into our cells, we create a poor environment for our genes, interfering with their ability to perform well.

Gene expression can also be altered by mind/body interactions like stress, emotions, and exercise. Stress and lack of sleep can release hormones and messenger molecules such as cortisol that can lead to diabetes, weight gain, osteoporosis, cognitive impairment, and damage to brain neurons. Exercise can counteract these effects by lowering levels of cortisol, thus preventing the same conditions.

There has been a great deal of excellent research that accentuates this point, especially work on identical twins, looking for concordance or discordance in terms of health. In one Scandinavian study, 44,000 pairs of twins were assessed to determine whether cancer was genetic. Researchers found that less than 10 percent of cancer cases studied were. The rest were environmental in origin, resulting from lifestyle choices such as diet and personal habits. Only breast and colon cancer showed a strong hereditary inclination.

We believe that locked within every cell is a healthier you. By creating a better environment for our genes, all of us can promote the optimal expression of these genes, resulting in more efficient and possibly even younger characteristics in our cells.

In conclusion: Most doctors are still treating your family history rather than you. But when we hear, "It runs in my family," we ask, "*What* runs in your family? Heart disease? Insulin resistance? Was yours a family that was stressed out, didn't exercise, and ate pork rinds for breakfast?" What really runs in the family?

We tell people that most of them inherited their parents' habits as much as they inherited their genes.

Still, doctors don't want to let go of the immutable gene myth. For many, surrendering to this myth has an almost fatalistic aspect— they're ready to throw in the towel before they see if they can really help you. They come from the model of suppressing and opposing illness instead of supporting health. However, we want to find out how your genes work and make them work better.

Sandy is an excellent example of the ability to change genetic destiny. A thirty-two-year-old woman who attended one of our Canyon Ranch lectures a few years ago, she approached us with tears in her eyes after she heard us say that people were not necessarily doomed to live out what seemed to be their genetic destiny.

Sandy was generally healthy and had two small boys, but both of her parents had died in their early forties of heart disease (within two years of each other). Sandy was petrified of following in her parents' footsteps and leaving her children motherless.

Sandy was also suffering from feelings of anxiety and powerlessness. She had consulted with numerous doctors, including cardiologists, and had good relationships with them, but none had really helped her. In fact, her anxiety level had prompted them to prescribe antidepressants and antianxiety drugs, which she was now taking.

Meanwhile, her doctors had run the usual tests, including those for stress and cholesterol levels. The results were fine—but this made Sandy even more uneasy, because they hadn't found any explanation for her family history, and she felt even more at the mercy of her genetic inheritance.

After talking with Sandy, we recommended that she have two additional blood tests that might offer some insight: those for her homocysteine and lipoprotein(a) (Lp[a]) levels. Elevations in both of these can explain an inheritance pattern of premature cardiovascular disease in someone without other apparent risk factors.

The tests hit pay dirt. Sandy's homocysteine level was 16, or twice as high as it should be, and her Lp(a) level was 120, which was four times the normal level. Both of these values might help explain her parents' disease—they likely also had elevated levels, a trait Sandy had inherited. However, both homocysteine and Lp(a) can be controlled with specific vitamin therapy. (Remember: Even though tests for homocysteine or Lp(a) levels are not routine, a great deal of research shows these two substances are independent risk factors for heart attack and stroke.)

Now there was something we could do to reduce Sandy's risk. We started her on therapeutic doses of folic acid, vitamin $B_6$, vitamin $B_3$, and vitamin $B_{12}$, and arranged for her to have her levels of homocysteine and Lp(a) rechecked in six weeks.

Six weeks later came the good news: Sandy's homocysteine level had dropped to 11 and her Lp(a) level was down to 65.

Sandy was thrilled to hear the news. For the first time she felt as though she'd thrown off the shackles of her unfortunate family history and had regained some control over her health. Eight weeks later her homocysteine level was in the normal range, at just under 8.5, and her Lp(a) level was down to 47. Sandy continues to take her supplements daily, and she no longer worries that she'll repeat her parents' medical history.

# MYTH 5: GETTING OLDER
# MEANS AGING

Ramona was fifty-six years old when she first came into our office. At the time she smoked, drank, and ate anything she felt like eating. A charming Southern belle, Ramona led a glamorous and active life, without any consideration for her health.

We don't often see such people at our door, but Ramona had sought us out because she had heard us give a lecture on osteoporosis, which made her aware of the risks her lifestyle was creating. She quickly told us, "I drink too much, I smoke, I don't take any calcium, and I don't really exercise"—which were indeed four of the major risks we mentioned in our lecture. Ramona realized that maybe, just maybe, it was time for her to start taking her health seriously.

Her hunch was correct. We soon found that she was in the early stages of osteoporosis, which meant that she already had substantial bone loss. Osteoporosis is not like osteoarthritis; you don't feel any pain until you break a bone, so it's not always obvious when you suffer from it. Yet osteoporosis makes your bones so thin that they become prone to fracture, meaning that you can be in genuine jeopardy without even knowing it.

Poor bone density is like a building in which the beams are thin and porous, or like a bridge with rotting arches; there are no supporting structures to hold up the bone. Imagine Swiss cheese; in fact, you can almost see the little holes in the bones.

After taking several of our diagnostic tests, Ramona realized how serious her condition was, and she was ready to take our advice. (She also turned out to have low blood sugar, and although she wasn't overweight, she had a low muscle mass. Most worrisome to her was that her face was wrinkling quickly.)

We asked Ramona to stop drinking, to exercise, and to take a total integrated bone-support formula containing calcium citrate (which is an absorbable form of calcium), along with magnesium, vitamin D, vitamin K, and trace elements including zinc and boron. We also asked her to eat soy, flaxseed, arugula (which has lots of calcium), and sea vegetables.

Ramona did exactly as requested and, after a year, returned with better bones—a 3 percent improvement in her bone density as measured by a bone density scanner. Three percent may not sound like much, but it's actually excellent. Few drugs claim better results.

Still, we were confident that Ramona could do even better, so we told her to work harder and to try some strength training as well. When Ramona came back to see us one year later, her bone density was 10 percent higher. And she had become a fanatic about strength training, working out four times a week.

"My body has changed," she bragged. "I no longer have those flabby, skinny arms, and all my friends are copying me—as usual. On top of that, my skin isn't wrinkling as much."

Just as Ramona's bones had been losing their structure and strength, so had her skin, which is supported by important connective tissue, such as collagen (when the supportive tissue and collagen become thinner, the skin reacts by wrinkling; oxidative stress and inflammation caused by poor diet, alcohol, and smoking also contribute to wrinkles). Ramona's skin tone and thickness improved as her bone density improved.

Ramona refused to stop smoking, however, and it was clear that nothing we could say would stop her. Frankly, we were amazed she could have achieved such significant gains and still smoke.

★   ★   ★

Yes, taxes are inevitable, death is inevitable, and aging is inevitable. But disease is not an inevitable part of aging. Getting older doesn't mean getting sick. We are all going to get older. But we are not all going to get sick—at least not in the same way.

It is even possible to become biologically younger while you become chronologically older. Aging is a measurable biological phenomenon that may be slowed or, in some cases, temporarily reversed.

It is true there's plenty of bad news concerning aging: You'll lose aerobic efficiency and muscle mass, your bone strength will drop, your sexual potency and desire will wane, your ability to regulate your body temperature will change, your basal metabolism (the number of calories your body consumes at rest) will drop; you will also become less sensitive to the effects of insulin, your cholesterol level will rise, and your body fat will increase. But these changes can be reversed, and to some degree they can even be prevented.

All of us want to die as old as possible feeling as young as possible; we want to be in perfect health until we're one hundred, then go to sleep and not wake up. That's not such an impossible wish. But to accomplish it, you have to work at it.

We like the statement made at one of our lectures by a sixty-five-year-old woman who exercises like mad, eats well, takes all her supplements, and has the body of a forty-year-old. Another woman said to her, "Aren't you too old to be doing all this?"

She replied, "I'm too old not to."

She's right. You have to work harder as you get older to maintain an optimal level of functioning.

Most of us think that aging is accompanied by decline because that's what we see. We are a society that supports the decline of the human body. Through the lack of physical activity, through the increased refinement of our foods, through the worsening of our diet, through mandatory retirement at age sixty-five, we create a more negative picture of aging than nature does.

In other cultures, where seniors are valued as wise and essential members of society, as keepers of knowledge and traditions, the aging process can be very different. But here we disregard seniors' talents, we lose interest in their lives, we place them in nursing homes.

Travel with us for a moment to Mexico, where the Tarahumara Indians have lived for centuries. These Indians are runners; rather than walk or ride a horse, they run from village to village. Living in remote and almost inaccessible villages, over the years the Tarahumara have become perfectly conditioned for long-distance running. They are celebrated for their endurance and are known to run fifty or sixty miles to hunt, to carry messages, or simply because it's enjoyable.

Here's the kicker: These people believe that the older runners are their best.

Not long ago a team of Harvard University researchers traveled to Mexico and recorded various physiological measurements from the Tarahumara, including aerobic capacity, fitness levels, and breath capacity. They found that, indeed, the sixty-year-old Tamahumaras were in better shape than the forty-year-olds, who in turn were better off than the twenty-year-olds.

The Tarahumaras know something that Western medicine is just learning about stable, long-term health: maintaining function, having interests, and keeping active are necessary.

Frankly, at Canyon Ranch we don't think that retirement at age sixty-five is a good thing. Perhaps we should do things in reverse: Start at age twenty with retirement, enjoy life, build a family, then at thirty-five go to work for the rest of our years.

Today there are remarkable members of our society who are eighty or ninety or older who haven't accepted the fact that they are going to be afflicted with illness.

Tom Spear is a 102-year-old golfer who plays eighteen holes three times a week and scores fifteen strokes less than his age. He won the fifty-five-and-over tournament in Calgary, Canada, when he was almost a half century older than the youngest participant.

Dirk Struik, a professor at the Massachusetts Institute of Technology and a figure of worldwide renown in the area of ethnomathematics (the study of mathematics in primitive cultures), continues to publish and lecture at the age of 104.

Jack LaLanne is quite possibly the fittest and most vital eighty-five-year-old on the planet. He has lived, breathed, and slept fitness and optimal nutrition since he was fifteen years old. On his seventieth birthday, as a testament to what healthy living and fitness can achieve, LaLanne arranged a demonstration during which he towed seventy boats with seventy people in them while shackled and handcuffed for a mile and a half, swimming against strong currents (not something we recommend for most seventy-year-olds).

One of the greatest American doctors, and the man whom natural medicine advocate Andrew Weil considers his mentor, was Dr. Robert Fulford. We highly recommend his book, *Dr. Fulford's Touch of Life*. Dr. Fulford wrote it as a ninety-one-year-old while he was still practicing medicine and successfully treating patients whom doctors one-third his age had decided they couldn't help.

Part of the problem is that conventional medicine deals with age in the same dismissive way as the rest of our society. Here's a joke we've often heard that isn't all that funny: A ninety-year-old man visits his doctor and says that his knee is bothering him. The doctor says, "What do you expect? You're ninety years old." The man says, "True, but my other knee is also ninety and it doesn't hurt."

Doctors seem to feel that if you're old, you should feel bad, and there's nothing anyone can do about it—except, perhaps, take pills, which often makes things worse. The elderly have been given so many medications over the last few decades that by the time they reach their eighties, they may be taking a dozen different ones.

Yet the older someone gets, geriatric medicine tells us, the less medicine they need. In the *PDR,* nearly every drug listed provides warnings for elderly patients, such as, "In general, dosages in the lower range are sufficient for most elderly patients."

For example, when older people develop swelling around the ankles, many doctors will put them on Lasix, a diuretic. But the problem is that most people who spend too much time sitting develop swollen ankles. Often this swelling may even be caused or aggravated by other medications (for example, calcium blockers prescribed for high blood pressure). If these people simply walked more frequently, they might not even have the swelling. But their diuretics, which can cause terrible dehydration, make it even harder to move. The result is an older person who's weak, tired, and can barely get out of the chair. If their doctors helped them become rehydrated by stopping their diuretics and having them drink more fluids, they might function again quite normally.

Beliefs, we are learning, can be self-fulfilling. In a 1979 Harvard study, researchers turned back the clock for a group of men aged seventy-five and older. The researchers brought these men to a retreat center and asked them to pretend it was 1959. The center duplicated life as it was in the late 1950s through music, magazines, and books; furthermore, the researchers told the men to talk about events of that time period—in other words, to be the men they were twenty years previously.

Acting younger had a profound effect on these men. Their memory and manual dexterity improved, they were more active and self-sufficient, they took responsibility for self-care tasks they had depended on others to do for them. Even aspects that were considered irreversible effects of aging changed. Independent judges reported the men looked younger; their fingers lengthened; their flexibility, posture, muscle strength, eyesight, and hearing all improved. Focusing their awareness on being who they were twenty years earlier helped these men experience their bodies as more vital.

In the book *Aging with Grace,* David Snowdon discusses the well-known study in which 678 Catholic nuns were observed for many decades to examine the aging process, particularly with regard to the brain. These nuns ranged in age from seventy-five to 106, and in their lives Dr. Snowdon found some important clues that could predict which people are most likely to be prone to Alzheimer's. The best predictor of good health at age one hundred included the presence of complex thought patterns, a result uncovered by the fortuitous find of essays and autobiographies the nuns had written when they first entered the convent decades earlier. The nuns who had written the most complex, descriptive, and detailed auto-biographies as young women were less likely to have developed Alzheimer's in old age.

In another project, David Morris, a seventy-five-year-old doctor at New York's Hebrew Home for the Aged, decided his patients were taking far too many drugs and started weaning them. His patients' health quickly and surprisingly improved, yet family members, staff, and even patients often fought with him over the decision. Many people were more afraid of being taken off a medication than starting to take it in the first place. Luckily, the Hebrew Home's chief of medicine supported Dr. Morris, partly because he agreed with the idea, but also because it was good business; the nursing home's drug expenses had soared throughout the 1990s—in five years, pharmacy expenses had increased by $1.5 million to $2 million.

In medical school we were taught that after the brain reaches maturity, it begins a slow process of decline. Once all of the neurons (nerve cells) had formed and the proper connections had been made, it was all downhill—every day, every hour, neurons were lost.

More recent research, however, reveals this is not the case. There is now a substantial and growing body of research that shows the brain can heal itself by growing new neurons and making new connections.

The main obstacle to the healing and regeneration of neurons is the presence of inflammation in the brain. Research now indicates that even if brain neurons are injured, if inflammation can be reduced or eliminated, healing and regeneration can follow.

Studies of the brain in the setting of multiple sclerosis provide some of this evidence. Research with MRI and PET scans reveals that even after damage to neurons of the brain due to multiple sclerosis, healing, improvement, and regeneration can and do occur, as documented by repeated scans.

Another misunderstood concept is plasticity, or the ability to repair damaged tissue. Part of staving off age-related decline lies in understanding how to measure and identify areas where the organ reserve is declining, and then to support it in a way that preserves that organ reserve, while compensating for the loss.

Everyone has a certain degree of organ reserve. When you were born, you were given much more than you needed in organ function, in every organ. You have more brain tissue than you need, as well as more muscle tissue, more kidney tissue, more liver tissue, and so on. For example, dialysis for kidney failure is not needed until kidney function drops to less than 20 percent of what is normal. (Fifty percent of your kidney function must have been lost before it even shows up on a lab test.) You'd have to lose at least 90 percent of your adrenal gland function before adrenal insufficiency would become evident. And as most men know, men remain fertile with only one testicle. Every organ has reserve capacity.

But most of us lose this reserve capacity as we age, due to cellular injury resulting from processes that include our five forces of illness. The symptoms of that loss are silent, however, until such a large number of cells are damaged that the organ becomes weakened.

Some of this is inevitable. But our hypothesis is that by examining the body's cellular and biochemical function, we can identify problems at the cellular level long before an organ becomes seriously damaged. By intervening before organ reserve is compromised, we can slow down its loss, and therefore slow the apparent aging of any organ.

That's not to say we can prevent or correct all of the effects of aging. But if we can identify problems with cellular function early enough, then the treatment is not surgery, chemotherapy, radiation, or organ transplantation, but rather changes in nutrition, targeted therapeutic supplementation, or changes in lifestyle and/or habits—treatments that promote the natural healing processes of the body.

The current problem is that traditional testing checks only for organ damage, and not for cellular and biochemical function. If you ask your doctor to check your liver function, the blood tests usually consist of measuring the level of enzymes produced by the liver. Yet these enzymes are elevated only if there is ongoing liver damage. So these tests only look for active liver damage, rather than liver function.

New tests are being developed to more precisely measure the functioning of the liver. An example is a challenge test, which assesses the function of the liver cells by "challenging" them with a particular substance. Testing how well the liver can process a certain compound, such as caffeine or aspirin, is one way to evaluate how well the enzymes and cells in the liver are doing their job. (New tests can also measure the liver's ability to antioxidize. When the liver's antioxidants become depleted, damage to the liver cells begins. Knowing the levels of antioxidant reserve, and maintaining them, can stop this damage.)

Another example: Let's say you have diabetes in your family and you'd like to know if you might be at risk. Most doctors would test your blood sugar level. Unfortunately, by the time the blood sugar level becomes abnormal, there has already been a significant loss of organ reserve of the pancreas. However, by using a challenge test (giving a load of sugar and measuring the insulin and blood sugar response), you can gain much more insight into how the pancreas is actually functioning.

In short, most people believe that our life span is the same as our life expectancy. It's not: The average life expectancy ranges from seventy to eighty years, but human life span may be as high as 120 years. And for most of us, our health span (how long we are healthy) does not equal our life span (how long we are alive). The promise and practice of ultraprevention is to create a health span equal to your life span.

## SUBMYTH: ALZHEIMER'S DISEASE IS UNAVOIDABLE AND IRREVERSIBLE

We say that Alzheimer's is preventable and possibly even reversible.

The current statistics suggest that one-half of all Americans will suffer from Alzheimer's disease by the time they're eighty-five. But such a fate is avoidable if we can identify and eliminate the underlying causes of the disorder before too much organ damage occurs.

Alzheimer's disease is a complicated, poorly understood condition. This is partly due to the fact that it does not have a single cause. "Alzheimer's" is merely a description of a brain that has become damaged and scarred. This scarring results from inflammation, which probably has multiple causes, including *ischemia,* or inadequate blood flow to the tissues. If circulation is impaired, the tissues being deprived of adequate blood flow start to become inflamed. Adequate circulation is critical to maintaining healthy, noninflamed tissues. So poor circulation is certainly a cause of Alzheimer's, and explains why people with atherosclerosis (hardening of the arteries) are prone to it.

Inflammation can also result from toxic exposure; common

examples include exposure to heavy metals such as lead or mercury, PCBs, or pesticides. Certain medications could also potentially trigger inflammation in the brain, including stimulants such as Ritalin, as well as the antidepressants in the Prozac family. Unfortunately, these drugs have not been in clinical use long enough to document the potential for late-onset Alzheimer's.

Additional causes of inflammation include chronic infections, allergies, trauma or mechanical injury, autoimmune conditions, obesity, insulin resistance, mitochondrial damage, oxidative stress, malnutrition, vitamin deficiencies (particularly vitamin $B_{12}$), elevated levels of homocysteine, and much more.

Any of these triggers may begin the process of brain inflammation. Therapies that block, reduce, or reverse this inflammatory process are likely to protect against and prevent Alzheimer's. This probably explains why researchers in 1997 found that a commonly used over-the-counter anti-inflammatory drug reduced the likelihood of Alzheimer's by 70 percent. The drug was ibuprofen. (That's not to say we recommend that everyone start taking Advil to prevent Alzheimer's disease. In the process of protecting the brain, you could damage your kidneys, liver, or stomach.) In 2002, researchers found that those who ate the highest amounts of dietary antioxidants reduced their chance of getting Alzheimer's by 70 percent.

If the problem is circulation, then we need to improve that. If the problem is toxicity, or free radical damage, or mitochondrial dysfunction, or malnutrition, or vitamin $B_{12}$ deficiency, those specific problems also need to be identified and eliminated. Tests for each of the conditions that cause inflammation are now available.

An example: Stan is a depressed, sixty-three-year-old overweight architect with an eating disorder. Each year Stan would visit us, lose twenty pounds, go home, and then overeat until he regained his old weight.

Stan has been successful in his business but not in his personal life—he recently married his third wife, and none of his previous marriages was happy. His current marriage, however, was in better condition. But Stan started experiencing episodes of transient global amnesia—a medical condition in which he forgot everything for a short period of time. He consulted a neurologist, who diagnosed him with impaired cognitive function.

When we saw Stan, however, we realized that he had tremendous risk factors for arteriosclerosis: his homocysteine levels were high, he showed signs of insulin resistance, his arteries were surrounded by calcium and were narrowing, and he had diminished cardiac function. He also had nutritional problems, including a deficiency of essential fatty acids and the B vitamins, as well as an inflamed and overworked liver. And, because of his impaired liver function, Stan could not process medications well. He also tested for high levels of mercury in his system.

To make matters worse, he was under chronic stress, which was one of the factors causing his depression. Unfortunately, when someone has chronic stress and depression, his or her adrenal glands (the stress glands) start overproducing the hormone cortisol.

Cortisol is one of our stress hormones. Under conditions of acute stress, cortisol can help the body to respond in a protective way. However, high cortisol levels for long periods of time are dangerous, leading to such problems as thinning of the bones, osteoporosis, diabetes, cataracts, high blood pressure, insulin resistance, weakening of the cardiovascular system and the immune system, and damage to the gastrointestinal tract.

What's important here is that cortisol has also been shown to damage the brain. Cortisol kills neurons, especially in a particularly sensitive area called the hippocampus. The hippocampus is crucial for the function of memory, as well as higher intellectual functioning. If your hippocampal cells are damaged, you will experience short-term memory loss as well as the loss of complex intellectual functioning. This type of brain damage can occur from chronically elevated levels of cortisol—chronic stress and depression, therefore, can be treatable causes of dementia.

Thankfully, research in nonhuman primates has shown that after removal of cortisol, growth and regeneration of the neurons in the hippocampus can occur. So the treatment and reduction of stress and depression may even reverse dementia caused by cortisol.

Stan admitted he was scared. His neurologist, he said, had told him to get his affairs in order. But we thought that we could arrest Stan's memory decline, and even reverse it, by targeting the problems causing the brain damage. In Stan's case, this meant dealing with his vascular disease and circulation problems, his insulin resistance, his chronic stress and depression, his nutritional imbalances, and the toxicity from mercury and cortisol—a long list, but illnesses are often the result of complex, not simple, situations.

We began Stan on an aggressive program that included an optimal diet, vigorous and regular exercise, stress reduction techniques, and a cortisol reduction plan that included meditation, yoga, and behavioral therapy. We dealt with toxicity issues by treating his mercury levels (through medications as well as an increase in his vitamin C, fluid, and fiber intake). We also supported and enhanced his liver function with specific nutrients, and reduced the workload of his liver by removing the chemicals, preservatives, heavy metals, and unnecessary medications from his life. And we put Stan on therapeutic antioxidants (to deal with his free radical damage).

Within a year it was all good news: Stan had lost eighty pounds, his hippocampus had grown, his memory had improved, his heavy metal levels were lower, and his oxidative stress, homocysteine, and cholesterol levels were normal. There was also a measurable reversal of arteriosclerosis.

When Stan went back to his neurologist, he told Stan, "My God!

How could you have done this?" It was the first time he had seen someone "recover" from Alzheimer's, and to this day he still doubts that Stan is anything other than a one-of-a-kind miracle.

## SUBMYTH: THERE'S NOTHING YOU CAN DO ABOUT ARTHRITIS

One thing is certainly true: Anti-inflammatory medicine does little more than cover up symptoms. Not only that, it can burn a hole in your stomach, your kidneys, or your liver.

Long-term use of these drugs may actually accelerate joint damage by relieving the pain of arthritis without addressing the joints themselves. When the sufferer doesn't feel pain in the joint, he or she is likely to overuse it, causing further joint damage.

Anti-inflammatory drugs also have the side effect of reducing blood flow to already damaged or inflamed joints, which may hamper the healing process within these joints.

Yet there's also a growing body of evidence showing that natural nontoxic treatments, including the previously discussed glucosamine and chondroitin, not only relieve symptoms but also reduce joint damage. A study in the British medical journal *Lancet* (January 27, 2001) looked at 212 patients with degenerative arthritis of the knee. This randomized, double-blind, placebo-controlled study (i.e., the study was scientifically correct) showed that the patients taking 1,500 mg of glucosamine per day for three years showed no significant loss of cartilage during that time, whereas the patients taking a placebo all showed progressive joint space narrowing due to loss of cartilage.

There are many testimonials that mirror the research findings about glucosamine and chondroitin. Take Sylvia: At seventy-two, Sylvia was a tremendously active senior. Aerobics, tennis, yoga, dance, hiking, and golf were all part of her life. Sylvia was in excellent health—fit, slender, and happy with her life. Her only complaint was that her knees kept her from doing as much as her head and the rest of her body told her she could do.

Sylvia truly hated taking medication, even though she had been willing to try the usual prescription anti-inflammatories. The non-steroidal ones, such as Advil and Aleve, upset her stomach. She had tried the newer prescription drugs Celebrex and Vioxx, but they seemed to cause her blood pressure to rise, so she stopped taking them. Meanwhile, her orthopedist had told her that she might need knee replacements in a few years.

Sylvia had heard of glucosamine and chondroitin, but her doctor had discouraged her from using them because he felt that not only were there no good studies on their effects, they might be danger-ous because they aren't regulated by the FDA.

When we saw Sylvia, she was very open to trying something new, so we gave her several of the research articles on glucosamine and chondroitin. She read them, and soon started taking 1,500 mg of glucosamine and 1,200 mg of chondroitin sulfate daily in three divided doses.

Three months later her knee pain and stiffness were completely gone, and she was back to playing tennis and golf. She was even ballroom dancing again. She felt so good that she'd begun giving her pet poodle, Maxine, some glucosamine and chondroitin, and Maxine's response was similar to hers. Neither of them, noted Sylvia, experienced any side effects.

## SUBMYTH: DIABETES ISN'T CURABLE

Diabetes, the fifth leading cause of death in our country, may exemplify aging better than any other condition. Diabetics tend to age faster than almost any other people due to the disease's wide-ranging negative effects; they suffer accelerated damage to almost all their organ systems.

An article in the May 30, 2001, issue of the *New England Journal of Medicine* showed that the chance of developing diabetes in high-risk subjects (overweight, middle-aged men and women who already had signs of impaired glucose tolerance, or those with the inability to properly process sugar) could be reduced overall by 58 percent through lifestyle changes.

In another study published in the *New England Journal of Medicine* (September 13, 2001), researchers looked at more than 80,000 women for sixteen years. They then compared the high- and low-risk groups according to lifestyle. The low-risk group included those who exercised; ate less saturated fat, trans fat, sugar, and foods with a higher glycemic index; and ate more fiber. The results of the study: Full-blown diabetes was averted in approximately 90 percent of the group that followed the healthy lifestyle.

And of course, by preventing diabetes, we can also reduce the effect of aging on all of the organ systems usually affected by this disease.

### SUBMYTH: YOUR SEX LIFE WORSENS AS YOU GET OLDER

No one, not even us, says your sex drive will improve as you age.

But you can still have good sex (and many people do) well into your eighties and beyond. Yet most doctors won't go near the subject. How often does your doctor ask you about your sex life?

We ask all the time, because we believe sex is important to health. Studies indicate that those with active sex lives live longer. As reported in the *British Medical Journal* (December 20, 1997), a ten-year study of 918 men between forty-five and fifty-nine years old showed that overall mortality was 50 percent lower in men who had orgasms at least twice a week or more, as compared with men who had orgasms less often or not at all. There also seemed to be a "dose response": That is, the lowest mortality rate was in the men with the most frequent sex, and the highest mortality occurred in the men with the least frequent sex.

The same is probably true for women. An article in *Gerontologist* reported that women's mortality over a twenty-five-year period was found to be inversely related to enjoyment of intercourse: the greater the enjoyment, the lower the mortality.

Another study, published by Swedish researchers in 1981, showed that sexual dissatisfaction was found to be a risk factor for premature death from heart attacks in women. The main reasons for this dissatisfaction were premature ejaculation and impotence in their husbands. The study supports the idea that sexual counseling, coaching, and therapy for husbands with performance problems may prevent heart attacks in their wives! It seems that in women, the quality of sex may be more important than quantity, although in men the reverse may be true.

We do know this much: When your life is rich with intimacy and sexuality, you live longer, you suffer less depression, and you look younger. Healthy relationships make for healthy people.

The best illustration of this may be those individuals who change partners later in life and find a new and increased pleasure in sex. A good example is Ed, a sixty-seven-year-old retired investment banker whose wife died of cancer. The marriage had lasted forty years, and the loss was extremely difficult for Ed. He admitted he had not had any sex for seven years, given his wife's illness. What bothered him more was that he no longer felt any sexual desire, which made him wonder if he'd become impotent. His doctor had diagnosed him with depression and started him on Prozac, which Ed felt was helping.

But recently, Ed met a fifty-five-year-old psychologist named Claire. Their relationship, which started slowly, was becoming more intimate, and Ed was concerned about his lack of sexual interest and his sexual performance. His overall mood was better, however, and he felt he was beginning to climb out of the deep depression that had followed his wife's death.

When Ed asked if there was anything we could do, we recommended two steps. Because antidepressant medications can reduce sexual interest, and because Ed's depression had improved, we discussed a strategy of slowly tapering off the Prozac under the supervision of his psychiatrist. We also discussed the importance of communication about sex in his new relationship. Ed was willing and agreed to follow through.

Six weeks later we spoke again on the phone. Ed reported that Claire was very open to talking about sex, and their conversations had improved their relationship. And Ed began to notice sexual interest again. Soon enough, Ed and Claire were having an intimate sexual relationship. What surprised Ed was that as they began to have sex, he found his desire increased.

Many couples find their sex life declines because it's the same-old same-old. It's not about aging physiology; it's about the aging of the relationship. For these couples, therapy should be directed at renewing communication about sex and introducing new sexual experiences while working on improving intimacy in the relationship. This process starts by simply talking about a sexual relationship, which often requires someone to be the mediator. Counselors and therapists who specialize in couples work are good choices, but every doctor has a responsibility to inquire about and to help foster healthy and high-quality sexual relationships for their patients.

Of course physiology still plays a role. But the male potency drug Viagra has changed the landscape regarding declining sex in older age, creating a sexual revolution for seniors. The rise of Viagra has also shown that physiological issues need to be addressed to promote an active sex life for men later in life. Although the drug may improve a man's erection, it does not as easily improve a man's relationship with his partner. Psychology and physiology must be addressed concurrently. And there are many more options available besides Viagra.

For example, Tom, a vice president at a large conglomerate, was about to retire because he felt he was no longer able to do his job;

his brain wasn't functioning as well as it had in the past and he couldn't make decisions as easily. But when he came to see us, he admitted his biggest concern was that he couldn't have sex with his new, younger wife.

He also related that he had become more sedentary, had gained twenty pounds, and was taking Zocor to keep his cholesterol under control. A few simple tests performed in our office showed that Tom had a moderate degree of insulin resistance. Insulin resistance can have an adverse effect on libido and sexual performance—high levels of insulin reduce the amount of available testosterone (through its effect on sex hormone–binding globulin, the protein that carries testosterone in the bloodstream).

Tom's treatment program was directed primarily at reversing his insulin resistance. We also asked him to stop drinking alcohol, and prescribed three natural products: ginkgo biloba, ginseng, and arginine.

Arginine is an amino acid that has an effect similar to Viagra; it raises the levels of a compound called nitric oxide, which is a substance found throughout our bodies that causes a number of important physiological effects. One of these is vasodilation, or enlarging of the blood vessels. Because of this action, nitric oxide can lower blood pressure and improve male erections. By taking arginine, men can do both simultaneously.

Six weeks later Tom called us with good news—he had lost eight pounds, he had put his retirement plans on hold, and his sex drive was almost too high—his wife was complaining because he now wanted to have sex too often. All in just six weeks!

Of course, we also encouraged Tom to talk to his wife about her sexual needs, and how his changes were affecting their relationship.

On the female side of sexuality and aging, the most important issue that confronts women is the change of life: perimenopause and menopause.

Very commonly, as a woman experiences the hormonal changes that accompany perimenopause (the four to five years leading up to menopause) and menopause (when a woman stops menstruating), her interest in sex may diminish. This drop in libido may also be accompanied by a degree of vaginal dryness, which can make sex feel less enjoyable, and a reduced intensity of orgasms.

These changes are primarily physiological, related to hormonal changes, although there is a significant emotional component as well. Women involved in intimate and communicative relationships tend to be more satisfied with their sex lives after menopause than women in difficult relationships.

The largest sex organ in the body is the brain—the emotional aspects of sex can be as important as the hormonal aspects. For example, although menopausal women often notice vaginal dryness, this disappears when there is adequate arousal. Even in post-menopausal women, the amount of normal vaginal lubrication is directly proportionate to the level of arousal. Intimacy, communication, arousal, and foreplay become ever more important for women in perimenopause and after menopause. For some women, supplementation with very small amounts of natural hormones may also help to maintain normal sexual functioning without incurring significant risk.

For example, Mary, a seventy-three-year-old widow, came for a consultation because she had begun a new relationship six months ago. The man she was seeing was her age and quite interested in having an active sex life. It had been a number of years since Mary had been sexually active; she had passed through menopause over twenty years ago.

Mary admitted that although she had little interest in sex at this time, she was concerned about her partner's needs and was interested to learn if there was any way we could help. We quickly assessed Mary's hormonal history and found that she might benefit from very low doses of hormone replacement with estrogen, pro-gesterone, and DHEA.

We started Mary on a very low dose of estrogen given in the form of an estrogen patch (transmitted through the skin), as well as small amounts of natural progesterone and DHEA, an adrenal hormone taken orally, which has been shown to improve libido and sexual function in postmenopausal women.

We also prescribed Estring, a flexible elastomer ring that, when inserted vaginally in a manner similar to that for a diaphragm, releases very small amounts of estrogen to the vaginal tissues and reverses the thinning and atrophy that can accompany menopause.

When we next checked in with Mary, she was happy to report that her relationship was going very well. Not only was her partner satisfied, she also felt a renewed interest and satisfaction with sex.

# MYTH 6: FAT IS A FOUR-LETTER WORD

Pete is a thirty-nine-year-old marathon runner. He's healthy, muscular, trim, and active, running ten miles six days a week. At five feet ten, he weighs 140 pounds. But despite his activity level, when we first met him, Pete was not truly healthy: His cholesterol level was 225, his HDL cholesterol was 25 (it should be over 60), and, at 225, his triglyceride level was also elevated (it should be less than 100).

Pete already knew these numbers, but his regular doctor had questioned him only about his family history (his doctor believed in the myth that your genes are immutable). Because it turned out that Pete's parents also had high cholesterol levels, the doctor told Pete that he needed to take medicine to lower his cholesterol. That was the end of the doctor's concern.

On the other hand, our first question concerned Pete's diet. It turned out that like so many other patients we meet, Pete had completely cut fat out of his diet. He ate only protein and carbohydrates.

What was Pete's treatment? One of our favorite prescriptions: fat. Yes, fat. But not the kind of fat you eat when you devour ice cream sundaes and chocolate cakes. Instead we recommended the fat found in olive oil, nuts, fish, avocados, and flaxseed.

Within two months, Peter's cholesterol decreased eighty points and his HDL improved dramatically. He didn't need to take medications. He just needed more fat—the right type of fat, that is.

★   ★   ★

Dietary myths are among the most common medical fallacies. Why did they arise? It's a long and sordid story, but political pressures have certainly played their part. For instance, the "four food groups" that most Americans know from the USDA (United States Department of Agriculture) nutrition pyramid were first conceived in the 1930s, when the meat industry, the dairy council, and the grain industry joined with the government to determine the country's diet. Reflecting their collective wisdom, a perfect meal was deemed to be a cheeseburger, French fries, and a milkshake, with ketchup as a vegetable. This was not a scientific breakthrough—it was a successful lobbying effort.

Even the newest rendition of the recommended USDA food pyramid isn't much better. And it's undergoing yet another revision—but unfortunately the organization is still under the influence of special interest groups. Industry still has a great deal to say about what the USDA says.

The RDA, or the recommended daily allowance, is another myth that arose from the wrong model of health and disease. The RDA system was based on what was needed to prevent the deficiencies associated with disease, rather than on a model to create health. Today, most people believe that meeting the RDA will help them achieve health. The reality is that just meeting the RDA will only stop you from coming down with a dreaded nutritional disease like scurvy or rickets. Other institutions have driven nutritional myths as well: the insurance business, the drug industry, hospitals, the HMOs, and so on.

Vitamins have long been thought necessary only in amounts needed to prevent deficiency (hence the RDA), but a review published in the June 19, 2002, *Journal of the American Medical Association* has shown that vitamins in excess of the minimum recommended amounts have a significant role in preventing chronic disease.

Regardless, the sad truth is that most doctors fall for these myths.

And given what we've heard from our patients, the advice they give is often as deleterious to the patient as it is helpful—especially that most common piece of advice, which is, "Stop eating all that fat!"

Science tells a different story. In 1999, a forty-six-month study on the heart from Lyon, France, looked at 605 people who had suffered heart attacks and survived. Some of these people were told to eat a Mediterranean diet; others were told to eat the American Heart Association (AHA) heart disease prevention and cholesterol-lowering diet.

The Mediterranean diet included fat from foods such as fish, olive, and canola oils; it also included a high number of fruits and vegetables, beans, nuts, seeds, and eggs, as well as some wine. And, it was significantly higher in fiber than the AHA diet, as well as in two important fatty acids: alpha-linolenic acid (a polyunsaturated omega-3 oil found in flaxseed, and canola and soybean oil) and oleic acid (from olive oil).

The results? The group eating the Mediterranean diet had 50 to 70 percent fewer second heart attacks—a result that has led to revisions in the AHA's guidelines for a heart-healthy diet. They even had to stop the study early because too many people eating the AHA's heart disease prevention diet were dying from heart attacks!

Here's more fat-related news: The most recent guidelines from the National Cholesterol Education Program (NCEP), published in the *Journal of the American Medical Association* (May 16, 2001), describe a new syndrome called metabolic syndrome (or insulin-resistance syndrome), and advise people with this condition to eat more fat.

The NCEP states: "In those with high triglyceride and/or low HDL levels, an intake of 30 to 35 percent fat may help avoid too high an intake of carbohydrate. This in turn may help to lower triglyceride and raise HDL levels."

And one more result regarding fat and heart disease: Researchers on a well-known project referred to as the Nurses' Health Study (as it focused on a large group of nurses) tested women to see if they should be reducing their fat intake. Doing so did not prevent heart disease. Changing the types of fat the women ate did.

Thus the quality of the fat is more important than the quantity of fat. Or, as another *New England Journal of Medicine* article (November 20, 1997) explained, "Replacing saturated and trans fats with monounsaturated and polyunsaturated fats is more effective in preventing heart disease than reducing overall fat intake."

The myth that fat is a four-letter word probably started for a simple reason: People figured that if they were trying to lose weight, they had to shed fat. And it seemed logical that if you were trying to lose fat, you shouldn't eat fat.

In 1988 the U.S. surgeon general set out to gather the data to prove that dietary fat is harmful. But after eleven years and four project officers, the project was disbanded, because there wasn't enough scientific data to support the expected forgone conclusion.

Says writer Gary Taubes in the March 30, 2001, issue of *Science,* "Mainstream nutritional science has demonized dietary fat, yet fifty years and hundreds of millions of dollars of research have failed to prove that eating a low-fat diet will help you live longer."

Still, over the last thirty years, Americans have tried and tried to cut fat out of their diet, decreasing fat consumption from over 40 percent to 34 percent of our calorie intake. But the consequences of eating some of the 15,000 new low-fat foods on the market have been disastrous. The proportion of the population suffering from obesity has surged from 14 percent to more than 30 percent, and more than 65 percent of Americans are overweight.

The problem: A fat isn't a fat isn't a fat.

That's because all fats are not created equal; there are many different types. The three main categories are: *saturated fats* (primarily animal fats); *unsaturated fats* (primarily from plant sources and from fish), which include both polyunsaturated and monounsaturated fats; and *synthetic fats,* which include the trans fats, or hydrogenated fats.

The basis for categorization of fats is a technical one, and relates to how many hydrogen atoms are attached to a carbon atom skeleton; the more hydrogen attached, the more saturated a fat becomes. Although most saturated fats are animal fats, some, including palm and coconut oil, are found in the vegetable kingdom. The more saturated a fat, such as butter or animal fats, the more likely it is to be a solid at room temperature. (Fats like vegetable oils and olive oil, which are unsaturated, are liquid at room temperature.)

Meat from land animals tends to contain saturated fats because these creatures are typically warm-blooded. Think of it this way: Fats are more fluid when warmer, so at body temperature, saturated fats are still flexible. Thus beef and pork have higher amounts of saturated fats than other foods.

On the other hand, the flesh of cold-blooded animals like fish contains predominantly polyunsaturated fats, which are more fluid at colder temperatures. If fish had predominantly saturated fats, the fat would solidify in cold water and the fish would die.

Range-fed beef cattle, although their meat has saturated fat, have lower concentrations than commercially raised, grain-fed beef cattle, which have 500 percent more saturated fat in their tissues. After all, you are what you eat, and that includes cows. Free-range animals munch on wild plants, so the content of saturated fats in their tissues is lower. Likewise, wild game such as caribou, elk, or deer have higher concentrations of omega-3 fats in their flesh because of the plant foods they eat.

What exactly is an omega fat? The "omega" classification refers to the chemical structure of unsaturated fats. As noted, unsaturated fats are those that are generally liquids at room temperature, whereas predominantly saturated fats (such as butter) are solids at room temperature. (The omega numbers 3, 6, and 9 refer to the locations on the fat molecule where the hydrogen atom joins onto it. It is just basic chemical nomenclature, but these simple differences have profound biological effects in the body.)

For optimal health, our bodies require a balance of omega fats. Deficiency of one or the other limits our ability to manufacture the full array of fats needed by our bodies for healthy cells, organs, and tissues. (Our bodies are normally about 15 to 30 percent fat by weight, depending on gender and body composition.)

Good sources of the omega-3 fats include: fish, flaxseed, omega-enriched eggs, organic canola oil, walnuts, brazil nuts, and sea vegetables. Good sources of the omega-6 oils include evening primrose oil, blackcurrant oil, borage oil, nuts, and seeds. Olive oil is the best source of the omega-9 fats—but don't forget avocados and nuts such as almonds.

However, omega-6 fats are much more prevalent than omega-3 fats. The optimal ratio of omega-6 to omega-3 fats in our diet is between 2:1 and 4:1, whereas the standard American diet has a ratio of more than 20:1. This means most of us need to increase our intake of omega-3 fats and reduce our intake of omega-6 fats. (Omega-9 foods generally should play more of a role in our American diet, and most of us should get the lion's share of our fats from omega-3s and omega-9s.)

Of all of the fats, our bodies actually require only two: *alpha-linolenic acid* (an omega-3) and *linoleic acid* (an omega-6). As with some vitamins, our bodies need these two fats but cannot manufacture them. By using these as raw materials, however, we can manufacture all of the other fats our bodies use.

Sources of the omega-6 linoleic acid include safflower and sunflower oils, and corn, soy, and canola oils. Sources of the omega-3 alpha-linolenic acid include flaxseed oil and blackcurrant seed oil. They can also be found in smaller amounts in certain nuts and seeds.

Deficiencies in these two essential fatty acids can cause dry, scaly skin; hair loss; slowed wound healing; easy bruising; and a goose-flesh type of eruption on the skin, usually over the backs of the arms or upper thighs. (Such deficiencies can also cause heart disease, diabetes, cancer, and depression.) Supplementing with the essential fats reverses these conditions.

While the saturated fats are more likely to lead to fatty buildup in the walls of our arteries, the unsaturated fats—particularly the monounsaturated fats and the omega-3 polyunsaturated fats—are less likely to do so.

Of all the fats, we find the so-called synthetic, or trans fats, to be the most dangerous. These man-made products are fats that have been altered chemically to produce new substances.

The reason the food industry created trans fats is that these fats are very resistant to oxidation (or going rancid), giving foods with high trans fat content a very long and stable shelf life. Trans fats include partially hydrogenated fats, margarine, and shortening; today they can be found in every aisle of the supermarket. You can keep that jar of Crisco in your cabinet for thirty years and still make a fine pie crust with it.

But just as bacteria (which make food go bad) have difficulty in digesting these fats, so do humans. The body doesn't have natural enzymes that can easily break them down. Intake of trans fats has been associated with increased rates of cardiovascular disease and cholesterol levels, as well as increased incidence of cancer and diabetes.

Here's the key to understanding the importance of fat: Intake of unsaturated fats is essential and critical to the functioning of every cell in our bodies.

Indeed, fat is good for us. Fat allows us to be warm-blooded. It provides us with insulation, as well as a highly efficient source of stored energy. Without fat, we would have to crawl out on a rock during the daytime to warm up enough to move about.

The cell membrane, which is the outside surface of every cell, is composed primarily of fat and the mineral phosphorus. This membrane, which forms the interface through which each of our cells contacts its neighboring cells, has important functions.

The membrane is semipermeable, meaning that it allows some substances across and into the cell (including nutrients from food, hormones, messenger molecules, and so on) while keeping others out (such as large molecules, sodium, calcium, et cetera).

The cell membrane also acts something like a battery. Our bodies spend a significant amount of energy just maintaining the "charge" of our cell membranes; this batterylike action is crucial for the functioning of our cells and for protecting them from breakdown and deterioration.

The point here is that the types of fats that make up our cell membranes are very important. For optimal cell health, the cell membrane must be fluid and flexible, rather than stiff and rigid. To allow for this flexibility and fluidity, the fats composing the cell membrane also need to be fluid and flexible. If the fats within our cell membranes are stiff and rigid, as happens when we fill ourselves with saturated and/or hydrogenated fats, the cell membrane becomes stiffer, less fluid, less able to perform optimally.

Guess what? The monounsaturated and polyunsaturated vegetable fats are some of the fluid, flexible fats. But no single fat or oil should be the only fat in your diet. Eating a balance and blend of the mono- and polyunsaturated fats is important for optimal cellular and general health.

Studies show that the proportions, or ratios, of certain fats in the diet have an impact on the level of inflammation in our bodies. Diets that are too high in the polyunsaturated fat known as arachidonic acid may lead to an increase in inflammation. Foods that are high in arachidonic acid include red meats, shellfish, and egg yolks.

As mentioned, the ratio of omega-3 to omega-6 fats in the American diet is lower than it should be, which may account for the high level of cardiovascular disease and other inflammatory conditions in the United States. In countries where fish intake is higher, rates of cardiovascular disease are much lower, and this may be related to the types of fats eaten in these places.

There's been a recent inversion of our diet even more dramatic than the way we switched from a hunter-gatherer society to an agricultural society. This is due to our practice of refining oils, which has increased the saturated fats and vegetable oils in our diets.

Back when humans were hunter-gatherers, our diets contained a 4:1 ratio of omega-3 to omega-6 fats. That ratio remained constant for eons, and it suitably reflects the makeup of our membranes. Diets rich in omega-3 fats are associated with lower rates of cardiovascular disease. Once we began to refine oils from plants, we switched to a high omega-6 diet, which accounts for the more than 20:1 ratio previously mentioned. As a result of our use of refined vegetable oils, we've changed the way our bodies work. This shift is making our bodies malfunction, causing inflammation, dry skin, and increased oxidation—some of the side effects of fat deficiency.

Today some well-informed doctors have started giving omega-3 fats to heart attack patients to reduce the risk of a second attack. Why? These fats thin the blood and reduce the stickiness of platelets (the tiny cells in our blood that initiate clotting). They also reduce inflammation, triglyceride levels, and blood pressure, and increase HDL.

After all, when our diet was brimming with these healthy fats, heart disease was almost nonexistent. Now it's the number-one cause of death in the developed world.

★   ★   ★

What happens to the body when the saturated fat content increases?

Imagine yourself miniaturized, traveling down an artery in your body, floating in your own bloodstream. Here you'll see a lot of red corpuscles carrying oxygen and carbon dioxide to and from the lungs and tissues. You'll also see white blood cells, the soldiers of our immune system, and platelets, the small cells that plug holes in our blood vessels if one was to spring a leak.

And you will see thousands of tiny, microscopic fat globules. Our bodies employ these globules to transport fats, which we use as a storage form of fuel, for the production of hormones, for the function of our immune system, for the growth and repair of cells in all tissues, and for many other purposes.

If all is well, these fat globules should travel smoothly through the arteries and not stick to the arteries' inside lining. If they do stick, due to thick blood, stagnant flow, or a sticky artery wall (or for any number of other reasons, all triggered by inflammation), then plaque growth begins.

As more of these fats are deposited (become stuck), they accumulate just beneath the smooth, protective membrane that normally lines the inside of the arteries. If this buildup continues, even more plaque grows. These plaques, which look a little like pimples, can erupt suddenly, just as a pimple erupts through the surface of the skin. This process is a catastrophic event, because as this plaque erupts, it causes damage to the smooth protective lining of the artery. This damage then triggers the process of clotting, and a blood clot begins to form at the site of the eruption. If this blood clot becomes enlarged, it can progress to the point of blocking off blood flow in the artery and a serious problem can develop, such as a heart attack, a stroke, or perhaps loss of circulation to a kidney, an arm, or a leg.

★   ★   ★

Now that you understand that fat is beautiful, you will come to appreciate it, as science is doing. Research is devising more and more beneficial uses for fat, including, strange as it may sound, as a treatment for depression.

At Canyon Ranch we have started prescribing fat to people suffering from depression, such as Marla. A thirty-nine-year-old in good physical shape, Marla exercised regularly and ate a reasonably healthy diet—but it was low in fat, as is common in many women who are careful about their weight.

Marla was married to a successful real estate broker, and had a stable and supportive environment. But she had recently experienced an acute manic episode, replete with extravagant shopping sprees—she once spent over $100,000 in a single outing.

Clearly she required immediate medical attention; she was given medication and by the time we saw her she had improved, but still was not well.

Recent research at Harvard has shown that supplemental essential fatty acids can improve the symptoms of bipolar (manic-depressive) disorder. This is based on the fundamental understanding that the cells of the brain normally contain high levels of DHA, which is also commonly found in fish fat, and that adequate levels of this type of fat are critical for healthy communication between brain cells.

A simple blood test showed that Marla's red blood cells were severely deficient in DHA and EPA, the essential omega-3 fats needed for proper brain development, mood, and cognitive function.

We then gave Marla high amounts of fish fat in supplement form. Soon her mood leveled out (as a side effect, her dry skin improved and her nails became less brittle). The fats in Marla's brain were not properly receiving the chemical messages of the happy mood chemicals. By putting these needed fats into her system, her brain became more receptive to these chemicals and could function better.

The April 23, 2001, issue of *Newsweek* reported on a man who had suffered a psychotic breakdown, becoming so delusional that he landed first in jail, and then in a psychiatric ward. Lithium didn't seem to help. His psychiatrist, Dr. Andrew Stoll, an assistant professor of psychiatry at Harvard, then recommended the man eat a quarter pound of salmon every day (while still taking his lithium). Six months later, Dr. Stoll was able to declare the treatment a complete success.

Please bear in mind: When you want to lose weight, you may think that getting rid of fat is the key. You see all that adipose tissue, or fat cells, accumulate on your body, and you think you have to get rid of it. This type of fat is very different from the fats humans need to perform essential body and brain functions.

On the other hand, don't rejoice because you have extra fat on your body—it doesn't mean your head is doing fine. Your love handles are merely a storage form of fat. They're not going to make you happy, in any sense of the word.

## SUBMYTH: MILK IS GOOD FOR YOU

The other night, after we gave a lecture in which we mentioned that we seldom recommend drinking milk, one of our guests jumped up and asked, "Well, if we don't drink milk, how are we ever going to get our calcium?"

The answer is: Plenty of ways. And milk isn't the best of them. In fact, the Federal Trade Commission recently asked the USDA to convene a panel of scientists to examine the claims in the milk industry's ads that feature the phrase "Got Milk?"

The panel found no support for the claims that milk improves sports performance or that it builds bone and prevents osteoporosis. They did find evidence of links between milk and heart disease as well as between milk and prostate cancer. And they pointed out the suffering caused by lactose intolerance for over 75 percent of the world's population, particularly among members of specific ethnic groups, including African Americans, Asians, Latinos, and Native Americans—who have been featured prominently in these ads.

Milk is nature's perfect food, the ads say—but only if you are a calf. The truth is that medical research has linked milk to many common and preventable health problems. It is a significant source of saturated fat in our diet, and has been linked to Type 1 diabetes, as well as chronic constipation and anemia in children.

In fact, the American Academy of Pediatrics recommends against feeding any milk products to infants less than one year of age. And milk may actually account for an increase in fracture risk, instead of preventing osteoporosis (see the *American Journal of Public Health,* 1997, vol. 87, pages 992–97, and the *American Journal of Epidemiology,* 1994, vol. 139, pages 493–505).

For many, milk is also the cause of allergies, sinus problems, eczema, and ear infections as well as a potential source of irritable bowel syndrome and digestive problems.

Think about it: 75 percent of the world's population doesn't drink milk, except breast milk in infancy. Where do they get their extra calcium? Nowhere. Most African women ingest little calcium—perhaps 300 to 500 mg a day—yet they rarely come down with osteoporosis. This is because they are not drinking alcohol, colas, or caffeine, or eating salt or excess animal protein—all of which can leach calcium out of your bones and into the toilet.

So if you're ingesting salt, sugar, alcohol, and cola, but you're not taking in a lot of calcium—rich greens, sardines, sesame seeds, nuts, or beans—you do need higher amounts of this mineral. The easy answer? Eat those greens, sardines, sesame seeds, and so on. (You can take supplements, too, but most of your calcium should come from your diet, because your body will absorb, and use, it better.)

By the way, there's more reason to be concerned with the effects of milk besides those related to milk itself. Consider the hormones, antibiotics, and pesticides found in milk that can also significantly impact our health. Bovine growth hormone, used to increase milk production, may increase the likelihood of breast cancer. And FDA surveys have shown that up to 86 percent of all milk samples contain antibiotics. On top of that, the fat in animal tissues, especially butterfat, stores toxins from the environment. These toxins are eaten by the cow in its feed and drunk in its water supply. Eating meat or milk are a fast way to bring these toxins into our systems. (Organic milk is better than nonorganic, but only in that it reduces the risk of antibiotics, hormones, and pesticides. It doesn't answer the other problems caused by milk.)

## SUBMYTH: EGGS ARE BAD FOR YOU

People have been dissing eggs for a long time. They think that cholesterol, which is found in eggs, in and of itself causes high cholesterol in your bloodstream if you eat them.

But here's a bit of news: Some time ago we read a study in the *New England Journal of Medicine* (March 18, 1991) about an eighty-eight-year-old man who ate twenty-five eggs a day. This man had completely clean arteries. We can't pretend his mental health was in good shape, because it wasn't. But the eggs weren't his problem.

The myth that eggs are bad for you took root because of the popular idea that cholesterol is the cause of heart disease. Researchers looked inside the arteries of people who had died of heart disease and found plaques that had cholesterol deposits in them. So it seemed as though cholesterol itself was the problem.

But science has since discovered that it wasn't the cholesterol at fault; cholesterol makes up little of our fat intake. And it would be extremely difficult to raise your blood cholesterol by eating cholesterol, since over 50 percent of all the cholesterol in our bodies does not come from dietary sources, but is manufactured in our cells, particularly in the liver and the intestines.

Our bodies make most of our cholesterol, because it is an essential component of every cell; it is a critical part of each cell membrane and also provides the critical starting point and building block for most of the steroid hormones in our bodies. These include testosterone, estrogen, pregnenolone, DHEA, progesterone, and cortisol.

Eggs are actually good for you. They contain folic acid, which helps to control our homocysteine levels; choline, which is an important component of our cell membranes, our nerve cells, and our brain tissue; and many more critical nutrients for building brain tissue, muscle, and cell membranes. Think of it this way: All the nutrients in the yolk are put there to create an entirely new life—a chick—so eggs have a lot of excellent nutrients in them.

A *Journal of the American Medical Association* article (April 21, 1999) on a study of egg consumption and the risk of cardiovascular disease in more than 117,000 people showed that those who ate the most eggs (six per week or more) had the lowest risk of heart attacks, and the group eating the fewest eggs (less than one per week) actually had the highest rates of heart attacks. In other words, egg consumption appears to guard against heart attacks.

## Submyth: All Carbohydrates Are Created Equal

While we're on the subject of fat, few people understand the relationship of carbohydrates to fat. Too many people, thinking they're eating a low-fat diet, are actually eating a high-carbohydrate diet, and that just isn't healthy.

What are carbohydrates? Simply put, they are a bunch of sugar molecules daisy-chained together. But for our bodies to be able to use these carbohydrate strings as energy, we need to break them down into their component simple sugars.

The speed at which this breakdown takes place determines how much sugar enters our bloodstream, and how quickly, after a carbohydrate-rich meal. That speed is important, because it has an impact on how much insulin we produce.

When sugar in our blood rises quickly, we make a lot of insulin. When sugar rises slowly, we make much less insulin.

As long as we're not diabetic, our bodies make exactly as much insulin as is needed to control our blood sugar within a certain range. If the blood sugar begins to rise rapidly, our bodies' response is to release more insulin in an effort to control our blood sugar level. But releasing a lot of insulin is not a good thing.

As we release more insulin, our livers become sluggish, our cholesterol and triglyceride levels rise; we put on weight and feel tired as well as hungry.

Over the long term, if excessive amounts of insulin are released regularly, our body develops a degree of tolerance, or resistance, to the effects of insulin, and we lose our normal responsiveness to it.

We then fall into a vicious cycle. As we become less sensitive to insulin, our blood sugar tends to run higher than normal, which triggers the release of more insulin, which leads to more tolerance, or resistance, which leads to higher insulin levels, and so on.

This process reveals the reasons why all carbohydrates are not created equal. Some carbohydrates can be converted to sugar very quickly, while other sources of carbohydrate are converted to sugar more slowly. How quickly any particular carbohydrate can be converted to sugar is indicated by something called the glycemic index of the food.

The glycemic index is a measure of how high your blood sugar rises after eating a fixed amount of carbohydrate. It is expressed in the form of a number that gives an estimate of how quickly that food is converted to sugar in our bodies. Glucose is the most common standard at 100.

The higher the number, the more quickly that food is converted. One of the highest numbers belongs to white bread, which has a glycemic index of 70. White bread can be converted to sugar very easily and quickly. Lima beans, on the other hand, have a glycemic index of 45, lentils 40, peanuts 20.

Here is a table from the *American Journal of Clinical Nutrition:*

# THE GLYCEMIC INDEX

### High-Glycemic Foods (60–100+)

Dates (dried) 103

Parsnips 97

Puffed rice cakes 91

Baked potato 85

Pretzels 83

Millet 81

French fries 75

Bagel 72

Popcorn 72

White rice 72

Pineapple 66

Beets 64

Whole wheat bread 60

Sweet corn 60

Boiled potatoes 60

### Medium-Glycemic Foods (40–60)

Bananas 58

Coarse whole grain bread 55

Mangos 51

Brown rice 50

Buckwheat 49

Grapes 49

Green peas 48

Kiwis 47

Carrots 47

Sweet potatoes 44

Oranges 42

### Low-Glycemic Foods (less than 40)

Plums 39

Navy beans 38

Pears 38

Yogurt 36

Apples 34

Chickpeas 33

Skim milk 32

Soy milk 30

Lentils 29

Peaches 28

Barley 22

Cherries 22

Cashews 22

Soybeans 18

Milk (full fat) 11

As you can see, foods like pasta and white rice tend to have very high glycemic indexes, because these foods can be quickly converted to sugar—usually because they are already processed or partially refined, so our bodies don't have to do much to convert them.

Simple sugars such as glucose, fructose, and lactose do not require much digestion; they are absorbed straightaway into the bloodstream. More complex carbohydrates, such as starches, require predigestion with enzymes, and are more slowly absorbed. Even more complex carbohydrates that exist in combination with fiber (such as vegetables, beans, and nuts) are absorbed very slowly, because they require more processing and digestion by our bodies before they are converted to simple sugars for absorption.

We often hear the terms *simple* and *complex* carbohydrates, but these are ambiguous and misleading concepts. The terms actually refer to the chemical structure of these carbohydrates; they do not explain their effects on our bodies, however, or even their availability to our bodies. We process the various simple and complex carbohydrates quite differently, and each has a different effect on our bodies.

Technically speaking, the term *simple carbohydrate* refers to sugar, of which there are several varieties, including table sugar (sucrose), milk sugar (lactose), fruit sugar (fructose), blood sugar (glucose), maltose (starch sugar), and galactose (a component of milk sugar). The term *complex carbohydrate* refers mainly to starches, which are chains of simple sugars; if the links of the chain are made of simple sugars, then the chain itself is a complex carbohydrate.

Whether a carbohydrate is complex or simple does not tell whether it is a good or bad carbohydrate to eat. A baked potato, for example, would be considered a complex carbohydrate, but we wouldn't rate it among the best foods.

As we've explained, the chemical definition has to do with the number of sugar units strung together; the simple carbohydrates have only one or two sugar units so linked, while starches are composed of simple sugars linked together in more complex arrangements.

Complex carbohydrates, like pasta, vary greatly in how quickly they can be converted to glucose, our blood sugar. Even simple sugars such as fructose and glucose are handled differently by our bodies and have different effects.

When it comes to diet, how quickly a carbohydrate can be converted to glucose is more important than whether a carbohydrate is simple or complex. Generally, the more slowly a carbohydrate is converted to glucose, the better it is for our health. (That's not to suggest that glucose is bad; it's just that the more quickly our blood glucose levels rise, the more insulin we release.)

One way to see how quickly a carbohydrate is converted to glucose is to look at the glycemic index of a particular carbohydrate. For instance, a rice cake has a higher glycemic index than table sugar because the rice is all puffed up, highly refined, and quickly broken down to sugar. So although it's technically considered complex, we're able to convert it to glucose immediately.

So ignore the concept of complex and simple! Instead, think about refined and unrefined. And think about the other characters in the mix: the fiber, the fat, or the proteins that in combination will slow the absorption of sugar into the system. Those are the important variables.

For instance, although a rice cake has a high glycemic index, if you spread almond butter over it, the glycemic index drops dramatically. This may seem paradoxical, but adding the nut butter adds some protein, fat (a healthy, monounsaturated fat), and fiber to the carbohydrate of the rice cake. The addition of protein, fat, and fiber to a food slows down how quickly the body can convert the carbohydrate to glucose.

There are a couple reasons for this. First, if the stomach has to digest some fiber, fat, and protein along with the carbohydrate, the process takes longer, the carbohydrate is digested a bit more slowly, and glucose enters the blood at a slower rate.

Second, the presence of fat in the stomach delays the emptying of the stomach contents into the small intestine. The stomach retains foods that contain fat longer to improve the digestion, or breakdown, of these fats. Since sugars are absorbed into the body from the intestines, if they enter the intestines more gradually from the stomach, their absorption into the blood is also slowed. So slowing the emptying of the stomach by adding fat to a carbohydrate meal can slow the absorption of sugar into the bloodstream.

This delay can be quite noticeable—people generally tend to feel full longer when the meals they eat include an ample proportion of fat. An empty stomach and hunger occur more quickly when a meal contains mostly carbohydrate with little fat or fiber. This may explain why people are much more satisfied with cheese and crackers than crackers alone.

Now some carbohydrates are not broken down at all, such as fiber, which is an example of an indigestible complex carbohydrate. Humans lack the enzymes needed to convert fiber to sugar (although other organisms do this quite well, such as some bacteria).

Still, even though we can't use fiber as a source of energy, fiber is an important nutrient, because it has a significant impact on the absorption of other, digestible carbohydrates. Fiber also has an effect on our digestion and elimination, and a major impact on the types of bacteria living and growing in our intestines, which can and do utilize fiber as a food source.

There are two main categories of fiber: soluble and insoluble. The terms *soluble* and *insoluble* simply indicate whether a fiber can be digested or not.

For example, bran is an insoluble fiber. It cannot be broken down by the body. This increases the bulk of the stool and the speed with which you eliminate waste, and may also cause absorption of toxins.

Soluble fiber comes most often from nonwheat types of fiber, such as from fruits or vegetables, and is broken down by the beneficial bacteria in your gut; these bacteria rely on soluble fiber as their own food source. Generally, the more soluble fiber in your diet, the more you promote the growth of healthy bacteria in the colon. These bacteria are considered beneficial because in the process of breaking down soluble fiber, they produce by-products that are important for our health.

For example, when acidophilus bacteria digest soluble fiber (e.g., from broccoli or greens or beans), they produce an important fatty acid known as butyrate. Butyrate, in turn, is a significant source of nourishment for the cells that line our intestinal tract, and this lining is critical for the health of our intestines, as well as helping preserve their ability to absorb food and eliminate waste.

Reduced levels of butyrate in the stool have been associated with colon cancer, as well as colitis (inflammation of the intestinal lining) and malabsorption (incomplete absorption of food from the gut). Since butyrate is produced by healthy bacteria in the process of digesting soluble fiber, eating more soluble fiber supports the growth of these healthy bacteria. This is a true symbiotic relationship: These bacteria are good for us and we're good for them, by providing them with enough soluble fiber.

So remember, carbohydrates come in many flavors and varieties. What's important to keep in mind isn't the simple-versus-complex argument you hear about so much in the media, but how quickly the carbohydrates are turned into sugar. The slower that process, the better off you are.

# MYTH 7: YOU CAN GET ALL THE VITAMINS YOU NEED FROM FOOD

Sara is a remarkable woman. Several years ago she was overweight and out of shape, taking too many medications for her ulcers and high blood pressure. But she recognized the perils of her situation and took steps to change. She began to watch her weight as well as walk every day.

But because her memory occasionally failed her, Sara was frightened that her brain was deteriorating. She had heard that food can affect brain cell function, and her doctor told her that eating a healthy, balanced diet might help (although he did not give her any specifics, and never asked her about her diet again). Still, eating well didn't seem to stop Sara's memory from becoming cloudy.

When she came to see us, we took some standard blood tests and found she had a very high homocysteine level. To rectify this, we designed a supplement program featuring folic acid and vitamins $B_6$ and $B_{12}$.

When we next checked in with Sara, she felt the supplements hadn't made a difference. We doubled her dose. That didn't seem to work either. We tried giving her four times as much. That still didn't work.

Not sure what else to do, we then gave Sara ten times the recommended amount of these nutrients. (There was nothing in the supplement program that would have caused any danger at this level.)

Finally Sara said that she felt a difference, and when we next conducted blood tests on her, we found her homocysteine level had indeed fallen back to normal.

It turned out that Sara had a unique need for certain vitamins. Without them, her brain was aging rapidly. And there was no way that she was going to obtain these nutrients from her diet, no matter how well she ate.

Yet when we tell other doctors that supplements are vital to our well-being, we hear any number of negative responses, the most frequent being something like: "Our ancestors have lived thousands of years without them. So we don't really need them, either."

Many of our ancestors also lived with poor vision due to a lack of glasses, with sun-damaged skin due to a lack of sunscreen, and with hypothermia in winter due to a lack of warm clothing. Do we really want to duplicate everything they had, or didn't have?

And as far as food goes, even if our ancestors' diet was perfect (which it wasn't), our modern diet actually lacks many nutrients common to our ancestors. This is due in part to changed farming practices and lack of organic matter in the soil (the source of many minerals and vitamins). Furthermore, many modern foods have been genetically altered for the worse (Indian corn has omega-3 fats, while modern, genetically modified corn does not). They've also been stored for prolonged periods before and during transportation (which depletes nutrients), then overprocessed and overprepared (which seriously depletes nutrients).

Furthermore, all the varying medications and over-the-counter remedies we take interfere or compete with nutrients for absorption. Considering all this, it's not surprising that more than 80 percent of Americans are deficient in one or more nutrients on a daily basis, at the level needed just to prevent deficiency diseases like rickets or beriberi. In fact, John Linenbaum at the Department of Medicine at Columbia-Presbyterian Medical Center has estimated that 10 to 20 percent of patients diagnosed with Alzheimer's have a functional $B_{12}$ deficiency.

And in a study of 494 healthy, middle-class people, as reported in the *Journal of the American College of Nutrition,* researchers found that more than 6 percent had a serious vitamin C deficiency, while an additional 30 percent suffered from borderline low levels of the nutrient. (Lack of vitamin C leads to scurvy, a disease generally thought to have been eradicated in the developed world.) But even with the minimalist RDA definition of our necessary intake, according to a recent USDA survey, more than 37 percent of Americans don't get enough vitamin C, almost 70 percent don't get enough vitamin E, almost three-quarters don't get enough zinc, and nearly 40 percent don't get enough iron. And nearly all Americans are deficient in the critical omega-3 fats.

Another reason that people didn't need to take vitamins in earlier centuries: They didn't eat as much. The more you eat, the more vitamins you need. That's because eating a lot of food equals burning a lot of food. Think of internal combustion—our bodies burn fuel like a car's engine. We ingest the fuel (food) and then we add oxygen; the oxygen and food are combusted, which gives rise to two outcomes: energy in the form of a chemical called ATP, and waste, which includes free radicals and other cellular products that have to be eliminated from the cells. This is similar to how your car engine works: It also produces energy, heat (dissipated by your radiator and cooling system), and waste (eliminated out the exhaust pipe).

One of the by-products generated by our cells while making energy is free radicals, about which you'll be reading more in Part II. But here's a brief explanation: Oxygen is a flammable molecule. If you're standing by a tank of oxygen, you don't want to light a match. The oxygen in our bodies is also flammable. It will burn tissue. That's why our bodies have developed a highly complex system to put out the fire of this excess oxygen.

Our bodies continuously make large amounts of antioxidants on a regular basis to quench the effects of oxygen. But sometimes we are depleted of antioxidants, or we can't keep up with the amount of oxidants we are taking in, and we get what is called oxidative stress, or excessive free radicals that aren't being quenched by the body's antioxidant system.

When this happens, you suffer from free radical damage, which is like a rust that starts on the inside of our bodies—in the cells themselves. So an antioxidant is something that fights the process of oxidation, just as Rustoleum fights the effects of oxygen on metal, or the way in which a little lemon juice added to cut apples prevents them from turning brown.

Food is a source of nutrients rich in antioxidants, including selenium, vitamin C, vitamin A, and the phytonutrients such as lycopene, xanthine, and lutein. (Phytonutrients are compounds found in plants with positive medicinal effects.) But food is also the biggest source of free radicals, manufactured by oxidative stress. This is because when the body processes food (specifically, when we convert food into usable energy inside our mitochondria), it releases free radicals that need to be quenched by our antioxidant system.

That's why so many research studies have showed that the best way to add thirty years to your life span is to eat less. The less you eat, the less oxidative stress is placed on the mitochondria—when they don't have to process as much food, they don't generate as many free radicals, toxins, and waste products.

Thus the people who eat the most food have the highest level of oxidative stress, and need the most vitamins to compensate.

We hear about vitamins and minerals all the time, but what do they actually do? Think of a car again, with its gas and oil. Food is like gas, but if you don't have oil in the engine, it won't run. That's the role of vitamins and minerals—they are like the oil. They help get your food processed through a host of biochemical reactions.

The real workhorses are the enzymes, or the little factories that change one chemical to another. Enzymes are proteins that have very important and very precise three-dimensional shapes that determine which chemical reactions in the body they can participate in.

We have thousands of different enzymes in our bodies. They are critical for all of the chemical processes that occur on a minute-by-minute basis. Enzymes help to digest and break down the food we eat. They help make energy. They are needed for growth and repair, for production of hormones, for detoxification, for proper nerve conduction.

For example, we need the enzyme called alcohol dehydrogenase to break down and eliminate alcohol from our bodies (it's found primarily in the liver). We need the enzyme ATPase to create ATP, which is the high-energy molecule our muscles and organs need to perform their usual functions. We need the enzyme transaminase to convert amino acids to fuel in the liver.

Many enzymes stop working if we don't have co-enzymes, or enzyme helpers. Often, elements such as zinc, selenium, molybdenum, chromium, vanadium, and so on may be required by enzymes to function properly. These trace elements must be obtained in our diets, because our bodies can't manufacture them. If our diet is deficient in these vitamins and minerals, the critical enzymes won't perform their catalyst function properly.

If your diet is deficient in chromium, for example, you may become resistant to insulin, since chromium is a necessary cofactor for enzymes that help insulin to function.

Or take the thyroid: Your thyroid gland produces two different thyroid hormones, called T4 and T3. T3, or triiodothyronine, is the active hormone that has many effects in the body (raising metabolism and body temperature; lowering cholesterol; controlling the speed of hair, skin, and nail growth; as well as many other functions). T4, the main hormone produced, is an inactive hormone that must be converted to T3 before it exerts its effects on metabolism.

T4 has four iodine molecules on it, and T3 only has three. In order for T4 to be activated so your body can use it, one of those iodine molecules must be removed chemically so it can become T3, with three iodine molecules. There's an enzyme called thyroid hormone deiodinase, which is a deiodizing enzyme. But in order for that enzyme to work, you need the mineral selenium (which comes in many foods, especially Brazil nuts, smoked herring, wheat germ, scallops, and barley). Without selenium, you're going to have a sluggish conversion of T4 to T3, and a whole host of metabolic functions will slow down.

Selenium is also critical in the prevention of cancer. A *Journal of the American Medical Association* article (December 25, 1996) reported that selenium supplements might be effective in preventing several cancers, including those of the lung, colon, rectum, and prostate. The exact mechanism by which selenium may prevent cancer is unknown, although we do know that selenium is very important in detoxification and in protecting our cells from free radicals.

In the liver (and in every cell) is an enzyme called glutathione peroxidase that helps recycle glutathione, the mother of all antioxidants. This antioxidant enzyme requires selenium to function properly. Without selenium, our antioxidant capabilities are sharply reduced.

Or consider magnesium, which is involved in more than three hundred enzyme reactions in the body. The depletion of magnesium can cause a breakdown in the body's chemistry. Magnesium is involved in critical reactions such as converting methionine (an amino acid you get from foods like meat) to SAM-e (S-adenosyl methionine, which is the newest of the natural drug remedies for depression). So without magnesium (which you can find in foods such as almonds, cashews, tofu, and kasha) the levels of SAM-e may drop, and depression may result.

Magnesium is involved in other chemical reactions as well, such as smooth muscle contraction, blood pressure regulation, and controlling the responsiveness of arteries to hormones. Magnesium is also critical in preventing the constriction of the small airways in the lungs that leads to asthma. It helps the energy production in all your cells, it's required in the metabolism of fatty acids, and it's critical for bowel function—without magnesium, you'll get constipation. This is just some of what magnesium can do; an entire book could be written on the subject. (In the meantime, you can increase it in your diet by eating lots of almonds, dark leafy greens, seaweed, peanuts, wheat bran and whole grains, okra, and, in smaller amounts, fruits.)

Even if you were somehow eating the perfect diet, you might still need supplements—because modern life demands it. Today we live in stressful environments; we eat processed foods full of preservatives, colorings, and flavor enhancers; we are exposed to pollution, pesticides, petrochemicals, and volatile organic compounds (VOCs). Our bodies require added supplemental nutrition just to help us cope properly with a toxic environment.

Research continually bears out this thesis. In a recent study of 609 children in India, it was found that taking just one multivitamin with added zinc lowered the rate of respiratory infections by 45 percent. *Archives of Ophthalmology* (vol. 119, 2001, page 1417) reported research findings showing that an antioxidant vitamin containing vitamins C, E, and beta–carotene with added zinc reduced the risk of developing advanced macular degeneration (damage to and deterioration of the retina, leading to vision loss and blindness) by 25 percent.

Supplemental folic acid and vitamin $B_6$ have been repeatedly shown to reduce the risk of cardiovascular disease, heart attack, and stroke, probably by virtue of their effects in lowering homocysteine. There are many more examples of research studies showing that supplemental nutrients can prevent, reverse, or slow many diseases.

★   ★   ★

Another problem that arises from relying on food alone for vitamins and minerals is that sometimes the foods rich in a specific nutrient are not necessarily the best conveyors of these nutrients.

Strangely enough, calcium-rich foods can actually impair your absorption of calcium. Dairy products, certainly high in calcium, are also high in protein, which has a calcium-depleting effect by increasing calcium loss in the urine. The largest distinctive component of protein is nitrogen, and when our bodies process nitrogen, it gets excreted in the urine, pulling calcium with it. So calcium combined with protein may not give you its full benefits.

Calcium-related problems can appear in nondairy products, too. Spinach and beet greens are rich sources of calcium, but they are also rich in oxalates. (Other high-oxalate foods include rhubarb and almonds.) When calcium combines with oxalate, it can form a crystal or a stone. People who have had kidney stones must be careful of oxalate intake, as this is the most common form of kidney stone.

When foods are rich in both calcium and oxalate, the stones form in the intestinal tract as opposed to forming in the kidney, and they block absorption of that calcium. So people who rely on spinach or beet greens for most or all of their calcium requirements may not actually be absorbing enough and should still take calcium in supplement form.

Sometimes the problem lies with the specific food's other contents. For example, phytates can interfere with absorption of many minerals and vitamins. Phytates, found in foods such as whole grains, cereals, peas, corn, rice, and pinto and navy beans, are similar to oxalate in that they bind with minerals such as calcium, magnesium, zinc, and trace elements in the gut. Once bound to these minerals, they are less available for absorption and use by the body. (Cooking and soaking reduces this effect.) Phytate intake may occasionally be a cause of zinc and other trace element deficiencies.

So if your diet is particularly rich in foods that contain high amounts of phytates, you may need to take mineral supplements between meals to assure adequate mineral nutrient status.

Despite our firm belief in supplements, there is room for caution. Don't take every pill bottle in the pharmacy. For the most part, the supplement and vitamin industry is unregulated. Certain unwanted ingredients may be present in your pills, such as artificial coloring, flavoring, hydrogenated fat, sugar, shellac, or even harmful heavy metals.

A recent *Journal of the American Medical Association* article (September 20, 2000) revealed that four of seven common calcium supplements tested had measurable levels of lead (depending on their source, which might include oyster shells or bonemeal). Why expose yourself to a toxic heavy metal while taking a supplement that is supposed to be good for your bones?

Or consider the new chocolate-flavored chewy calcium "treats" that thousands of women are now taking. Unfortunately, these calcium chews also contain hydrogenated fats, sugar (in the form of high-fructose corn syrup), and artificial flavorings. In addition, the calcium used is in the form of the more poorly absorbed calcium carbonate, making the chews a so-so proposition.

Furthermore, you can take too much of certain vitamins and supplements. If most of your calcium intake is diet-related, even in high doses, you're fine, but be careful if it comes from supplements, particularly if calcium carbonate is the source. An excess of calcium carbonate taken through a supplement can lead to kidney stones. This is the main reason we recommend taking calcium citrate instead. This strategy actually reduces the risk of kidney stones, and is a much safer, preferable way of getting extra calcium.

And some of the herbal supplements are downright dangerous; they are often grown in countries with no controls. Herbal supplements grown or manufactured in countries such as China or India may have measurable levels of mercury or arsenic. Soils in China are highly contaminated with mercury. No oversight, analysis, or government regulation of these products is required, so it's hard to know if any specific product is clean and safe. Reports of Chinese herbs actually containing prescription medications, including stimulants, steroids, or sedatives, are not uncommon.

But problems with supplements and vitamins are not limited to foreign countries. In fact, even in the United States, independent testing has repeatedly shown that many vitamins and supplements do not contain the doses, or even the ingredients, listed on the labels.

It's hard for consumers to know that they're actually getting exactly what—and only what—they paid for. We recommend the following precautions:

• Consider buying only from companies that will provide results of independent laboratory assays of their products.

• Be extra cautious with products grown or manufactured in foreign countries, particularly China and India.

• Look for results from independent labs, such as data found on www.consumerlab.com, for content and purity of supplements.

• Be cautious of supplements that contain unwanted ingredients such as sugars, fats, lactose, gluten, dyes, artificial flavorings or colors, glazes, binders, fillers, flow agents, or hydrogenated oils.

• In 2002, a government organization called the United States Pharmacopeia (USP) started a voluntary quality-assurance program for dietary supplements. Look for the USP mark, as it will indicate that the supplement manufacturer has developed a quality-control system to ensure that its supplements contain the ingredients and potency declared on the label, meet requirements for limits on contaminants, and comply with the various government rules for nutritional supplements.

★   ★   ★

Despite our poor diets, why do so many doctors doubt the value of supplements? In part because doctors tend to be skeptical; you have to show me proof, they say, and there isn't enough in all areas for all vitamins—too few studies have been completed. After all, why should the large drug companies fund efforts to look at the effects of folic acid when they can't patent it, or even produce it at the kind of profit they can make from their own drugs? Because they can't own them, they don't sponsor research on vitamins.

It's also difficult to conduct these studies. They require a great many people; they must take place over long periods of time, as long as twenty-five years or more; and they are expensive. The kind of money needed for this isn't available, unless the government is willing to step in (and the government does sponsor nearly all of the nutritional research, through the National Institutes of Health).

Yet modern medicine is willing to use vitamin therapy regularly in certain instances, such as using a magnesium IV to lower blood pressure and prevent seizures in pregnant women—but this is not thought of as nutritional therapy.

On the other hand, we practice nutritional therapy regularly. Take the case of Joan, a thirty-one-year-old investment banker. Joan had a fair complexion and was quite attractive, but when we first met her, she looked somewhat pasty and puffy in the face.

Joan had lived a life full of allergies. She was always vigilant. If she ate the wrong food or drank the wrong water, she came down with hives, eczema, or scaly dry skin. She also suffered from frequent colds, and her whole immune system seemed to be sleeping on the job.

She had seen the best doctors in her home city, as well as the best alternative practitioners. Still, no matter what diet she tried, or what therapies she endured, she seemed to get worse and worse.

When we met Joan, she was eating intelligently—lots of vegetables, beans, whole grains, and some lean animal foods; she avoided meat, dairy, sugar, coffee, and alcohol. Still she suffered.

After reviewing her lab tests, we noticed a few clues that seemed to have been previously overlooked. First, Joan's white blood cell count was very low; second, a liver enzyme called alkaline phosphatase was also very low in every blood test she had had over the years.

Most doctors pay attention to this test only when its result is high, indicating bone or liver disease. But what most doctors don't know is that this enzyme depends on zinc, and low levels correlate with zinc deficiency.

Over 70 percent of Americans are deficient in zinc, a mineral critical for healthy immune functioning (that's why evidence supports the theory that sucking on a zinc lozenge shortens the duration of a cold).

We gave Joan a little-known test called the zinc taste test. Since zinc is responsible for our sense of taste, drinking a solution with zinc can indicate zinc deficiency if a person cannot sense it, because normally it tastes like dirty metal.

To Joan, however, the solution tasted okay, which was a pretty good clue that she was zinc-deficient. When we double-checked, we indeed discovered a low blood zinc level.

After taking zinc for ten weeks (as well as eating zinc-rich foods such as eggs and wheat germ), and helping her immune system recover through our ultraprevention program, Joan shed all her allergies. Four years later she is still doing great. In fact, six months after we treated her, she became pregnant and now is planning for a second child.

Despite her otherwise excellent diet, Joan's body was missing a key nutrient that she apparently needed in greater amounts than she could obtain from her food, both because of previous stresses that caused her to lose zinc, and because of her genetic predisposition to her allergies.

A good diet often isn't enough to meet all our needs, needs that are particularly complex and challenged by our lifestyles, stress, environmental toxins, medications, and more.

## SUBMYTH: FOOD HAS NOTHING TO DO WITH YOUR HEALTH

Believe it or not, this myth is still pervasive among health professionals. They don't seem to believe that the food you ingest has an effect on your body. They may feel you shouldn't eat a high-fat diet, or they may suggest you eat less, but even when talking about the latest guidelines from the National Cholesterol Education Program, they will tell you to forget about diet and proceed straight to the drugs. "Take Lipitor," they'll say. "Take Lopid."

Most doctors don't think of food as remedial. They think of it as illness-causing, giving rise to heart disease, high blood pressure, or stroke. These naysayers' major argument is that food can't possibly affect your health because your system breaks down food in the same way: All fats are broken down into fatty acids, all proteins are broken down into amino acids, all carbohydrates are broken down into sugar. If all food turns into the same basic components, it can have no effects.

We say food is not just for energy and supplying the body with building blocks for growth and repair (the process of which is still not completely understood). It is also a source of information that communicates directly with your genetic material and, in many cases, can cure illnesses (or cause them). Foods that can harm and heal are well established in the medical literature, but are still not appreciated by most physicians.

This theory is what's known as evolutionary symbiosis: Humans have co-evolved with certain plants in a way that is beneficial for both species. We have cultivated these plants—such as grains, soy, and cruciferous vegetables—because over time we have recognized that they are good for us. And we are good for them, too, because by cultivating them we ensure their long-term survival.

Numerous cultures have recognized the beneficial health effects of these crops, and now even Western science has identified many of the healthful phytonutrients found within them.

For example, cruciferous vegetables (such as cauliflower and cabbage) contain the compounds known as sulfurophanes, isothio-cyanates, and indole-3-carbinol. All three can activate beneficial functions in the body, can improve detoxification by the liver, and can activate certain liver enzymes such as glutathione-S-transferase, which helps your body detoxify from pollution and toxic waste. They can also help neutralize cancerous compounds, support the liver's ability to process hormones, and reduce the carcinogenic estrogens produced by the liver.

Lignans, which are present in flaxseed (as well as other seeds, grains, and beans), have specific properties that affect steroid hormones' metabolism in the body. We used to think lignans were inert and valueless compounds, but now we see they can be powerful agents of healing and cancer prevention by promoting anticancer hormones.

Further examples of important healthy phytonutrients include catechins and epigallactocatechins (found primarily in green tea), which have anticancer properties and can enhance liver detoxification, lower cholesterol, and help regulate blood sugar. Compounds in soy and red clover known as isoflavones (such as genistein and daidzein) lower cholesterol and activate anticancer enzymes.

More of these healthy phytonutrients are being discovered every day, and substantial ongoing research has been identifying and purifying many of these compounds for potential use as medications to treat various conditions.

Another fact shattering the myth that all foods are broken down similarly: The way carbohydrates, fats, and protein are packaged for consumption is of vital importance. A carbohydrate delivered in the form of a bean has physiological effects different from one delivered in the form of white sugar: namely, the speed with which it is turned into sugar (as discussed in the previous myth).

Let's say you eat two isocaloric meals (or two meals with the same number of calories), one in the form of a highly refined grain, like white bread, and the other in the form of whole wheat bread.

The white bread is absorbed into your bloodstream much faster than the whole wheat bread, which means that your blood sugar rises more quickly. When that happens, your pancreas releases more insulin, which then has subsequent effects on the level of cholesterol in your blood, as well as the level of triglycerides, cortisol, and the degree of inflammation in your system.

The same is true for proteins—like fats, not all proteins are created equal. Proteins are complicated molecules made up of those basic building blocks called amino acids, and the balance of amino acids is important. If you think of a protein as a chain, then the amino acids are the links. When the amino acids are out of balance, people are prone to certain conditions such as depression, inflammation, and cardiovascular disease.

For example, as mentioned, the amino acid known as homocysteine can be dangerous. High levels of homocysteine are associated with premature heart attacks, dementia, cancer, and stroke. Certain proteins, such as those found in animal proteins, tend to raise the level of homocysteine, whereas the proteins in vegetables, containing different amino acids with different amino acid structures, do not raise homocysteine. Thus an excess of animal protein in the diet may cause harm, whereas consuming many plant proteins won't.

Furthermore, an animal protein such as steak contains certain amino acids that are more acidic than amino acids that come from plant proteins. The body has to compensate for that acidity, and one way it does that is by pulling calcium out of the bones, because calcium neutralizes the acidity. But the side effect of having the calcium pulled off your bones is that you're left with weaker bones.

Food is not simply a source of fuel to be digested down to its basic components and burned for energy or used for growth and repair. Food is also a source of information that has powerful physiological effects on our bodies.

## Submyth: One Multivitamin Is the Right Dose for Everyone

That's like saying one suit fits all. It doesn't. What's right for one person is not necessarily right for another. People need different blends of nutrients. Testing may be helpful in this regard. Our tests have shown that our cowriter, Gene Stone, needs extra chromium and vanadium. His carbohydrate metabolism is impaired and requires a special combination of dietary changes, fiber, phytonutrients, and nutritional supplements to correct that. Other people may need extra gamma-linolenic acid or lipoic acid, or inositol or zinc or $B_6$ (pyridoxine). Perhaps you need antioxidants, while someone else needs vitamin D, or magnesium, or manganese.

Modern medical doctors tend to think they are treating large groups of people at once. They aren't. They are treating one person at a time. As Roger Williams, the biochemist who coined the phrase "biochemical diversity," said, "Statistical humans are of little interest; nutrition is for real people."

Also important to keep in mind: Supplemental needs vary over time. What was right for you when you were twenty years old is probably wrong for you at age fifty. In fact, in just six months your vitamin needs may vary.

Your supplement requirements depend on your diet, your activity level and intensity of exercise, your habits, your substance use, as well as any changes in your weight, your age, your medications, and your stress level. Since these variables change, your supplement program should change, too.

# PART II

# Ultraprevention: Controlling the Five Forces of Illness

Human life, particularly in health and disease, is the result of countless independent forces impinging simultaneously on the total organism and setting in motion a multitude of interrelated responses.
—Rene Dubos, French-American bacteriologist

You don't have to wait until you are sick to get well.
—Us

# ULTRAPREVENTION AND
# THE FIVE FORCES OF ILLNESS

Now we want to talk to you about the system we practice at Canyon Ranch. All you have to do is go out and eat one leafy green vegetable a day. That's it! In fact, you don't even have to eat one of those magnificent vegetables. You can just think about one every day. If you do, you will never come down with a serious illness, your sex life will improve 200 percent, you will lose all your excess fat, and you will meet an attractive stranger, take a long voyage, and find the solution for world peace.

If only it were so easy.

It's not. All those books promising that your life will be golden if you do just one thing, or eat just one food, or exercise in one particular way, aren't worth the paper they are printed on. Such formulas are, in fact, myths no better than all those other myths you've been reading about—myths that reflect our basic desire for simplicity in the face of reality.

The fact is, the human body is complicated. The human system has evolved over hundreds of thousands of years. There is no one magic bullet that will shoot down all your health issues.

We believe, however, that once you stop falling for the myths of modern medicine, and once you begin adopting the recommendations contained in our system, you will be on your way to a future of better health.

That part of it is indeed simple.

We have named the approach we use at Canyon Ranch *ultraprevention*. A new paradigm of well-being, ultraprevention is a system of thought, evaluation, and treatment derived from the scientific study of health. Unlike most medical practices today, ultraprevention is based on remarkable truths uncovered by researchers over the last few years. These truths provide tremendous insight into our health and give us a basic framework that explains and unites the processes of health and illness, whether a person has anything from cancer to heart disease, stroke to high blood pressure, kidney disease to attention deficit disorder, and so on.

In all these diseases common forces can be found years, or even decades, before each ailment has progressed far enough to be diagnosed. And by addressing these forces, ultraprevention can prevent rather than simply detect or diagnose.

These forces are:

- Malnutrition, or sludge
- Impaired metabolism, or burnout
- Inflammation, or heat
- Impaired detoxification, or waste
- Oxidative stress, or rust

We believe that every person who pays attention to these forces will enjoy better health. Our program isn't just about getting better when you feel ill—it's about staying better so you don't have to feel ill at all.

Today many doctors talk about early detection as the cornerstone of prevention. But true prevention has to start long before detection can occur. This is because patients are not an ambulatory collection of separate organs and various conditions. Everything in the body is related. Imbalances or dysfunctions in one system lead to added stresses in the other systems. When these stresses and imbalances tax the organ reserve of any system, symptoms and illness result.

For example, if a problem develops in your intestines, added strain will be placed on your immune system, which can lead to immunological problems such as arthritis, hepatitis, skin conditions, asthma, or eye inflammation, and that intestinal stress also puts added strain on the liver, which can affect the blood and the brain.

Remember the old song, "The thighbone's connected to the hipbone, the hipbone's connected to the tailbone . . ."? There was more truth to that song than the writers may have known. Just as no organism can exist in isolation, neither can a body system. Each system is interdependent; the cardiovascular system with the immune system with the gastrointestinal system with the nervous system with the endocrine system with the musculoskeletal system, and so on.

Yet if you were to approach most doctors and say, "I feel like I'm getting arthritis in my hands, and when I eat pizza I get gas, and on top of that I seem to have come down with this weird skin rash," they may respond that they can only deal with one problem at a time. In our approach, however, these conditions serve as clues that, viewed as part of a larger picture rather than unrelated snapshots, provide us with information about your overall situation.

Most doctors don't try to put the clues together to form a big picture. It's as if Sherlock Holmes walked into a room, saw his first clue, and then refused to look any further. But, Dr. Watson asks, "What about these clues over here?" "Shush," says Sherlock, "stop confusing me with all those extra facts."

Let's say you wake up one morning and you're short of breath, with chest pains shooting down your arm—you may well think you're having a heart attack and go to the emergency room. And sure enough, the diagnosis is a heart attack. The treatment will be difficult, and the condition is serious.

But consider: This heart attack didn't just occur this morning. It was preceded by decades of plaque buildup caused by oxidation (or rusting) of fats in the bloodstream, which became deposited in the wall of the artery, followed by activation of the immune system leading to inflammation (or heat) in the wall of the artery, aggravated by (the sludge of) malnutrition, and tipped over by the resulting stress on the detoxification (waste) system, which finally made one of those plaques break open and rupture, causing a clot to form that in turn caused your heart attack.

A similar lengthy chain of events could lead to diabetes: a certain predisposition, coupled with burnout of energy production in cells, caused by the effects of insulin resistance, which leads to the heat of inflammation and the rust of oxidative stress, in turn accelerated by the sludge of an improper diet.

In fact, a similar chain reaction occurs with all common illnesses. The beginnings of these diseases are like the first in a long line of dominoes to fall in a reaction that may take years to complete, eventually ending with the diagnosis of a preventable illness.

Those first dominoes fell long before the problem occurred in a noticeable way. Looking for those first dominoes is what ultraprevention is about. Or as we say to our patients, "Let's find those first dominoes and pick them up before the whole chain has a chance to fall down."

That's why, even though the term *ultraprevention* has the word *prevention* in it, it works wonderfully at the treatment end of our medical practice, too.

Let's say somebody already has a disease, and we know which dominoes led to the development of that disease. Our system treats that disease—and reverses it. After all, the human body can right itself, if given the chance to do so.

Most conventional doctors don't seem to believe that. There's no particular reason why they should. These doctors spent many years attending medical school, doing their residency, and taking courses in continuing medical education, where they learned one major skill: how to diagnose.

As mentioned, the problem is that you may not be diagnosable. Think about going to see your doctor when you feel fine. Your doctor will ask, "Why are you here?" Try saying, "I just want to know if I can do more to make me stay great."

See if your doctor doesn't think you're crazy. If you don't have a symptom, he can't diagnosis a disease. And if there's no disease, there's no treatment.

Remember: The entire medical billing system requires a diagnosis. This means the doctor's thinking process often ends right there, with the diagnosis.

But we believe that diagnosis marks the *beginning* of the thinking process. It allows us to ask new questions, to understand new relationships, to go deeper into the interconnections of elements of patients' lives that have preceded illness. We seek the triggers of those illnesses, and explore how they manifest as symptoms.

Because the symptoms are warning signs, they're really clues to a much deeper process that we want to understand. We want to know what was going on before the symptoms occurred. Symptoms are the smoke; they're not the fire.

The crux of our system is this: If you look for the telltale signs of serious conditions years before a disease may be diagnosed, and you address these signs, you can prevent the development of the disease.

For example, your homocysteine level may be somewhat elevated, and that causes no symptom, but there will be a result—a stroke, or Alzheimer's, or a heart attack, or cancer—sometime in the future. Likewise, if your insulin levels are high for twenty years, you may not feel a lot of symptoms, except perhaps being tired after meals or getting a little fat around the middle.

Still, those are real problems that have serious consequences. Most doctors won't take on this discussion. But in ultraprevention, it's essential.

True health is not the absence of disease. Just because you have not been diagnosed with a disease doesn't mean that your body is functioning well.

But if you wait until a disease has progressed to the stage when a doctor can find it and diagnose it, that disease may already have advanced to a potentially fatal level.

If this is all so obvious, why doesn't every doctor know it? One of the most common questions we hear is, "How come my doctor hasn't told me about these issues?"

The answer is because few doctors have any experience in it. We do. Our ideas come directly from our work. We are not specialists, we are not researchers—we're practicing physicians and we have acquired a great deal of experience in our system of medicine by virtue of our great fortune in working at Canyon Ranch, where we see patients every day. Most of our patients are highly motivated to explore the effects of diet, lifestyle, and nutrition on their health and sense of well-being. We have, in effect, an ongoing laboratory. We are able to reflect on, and learn from, our patients' responses and their histories.

This fortuitous situation has only reinforced our sense of how different each patient is from the next, as we often see similar disorders for which the treatment will work well in one person, and not as well in another. (Yes, sometimes we take a wrong turn—but much more often we take a right turn, and frequently we take turns that no one else has taken before.)

Furthermore, unlike most doctors, we have the time to keep up with research as it is published, and to incorporate new discoveries into our work. Thus our medical model is information-based, and is always ready and able to take in new information. This elasticity allows us to constantly update our predictive model for assessment and treatment of each patient, integrating the best of conventional, alternative, and new scientific models, which in turn allows us to offer a brand of medicine that we believe is actually good for our patients.

Some doctors and patients have asked us if *ultraprevention* isn't simply another word for integrative health or holistic health.

The answer is no. We feel integrative medicine is too often a patchwork quilt of disparate systems fused together in an almost haphazard way, hoping for some kind of benefit: Swallow this herb, take this acupuncture treatment, try this healing touch. But all of those treatments in themselves are separate systems, representing worldviews that don't necessarily blend well. We think of that kind of practice as less an integrative philosophy than an "associated" one: Its various elements may be related, but they don't necessarily derive from the kind of common concepts that provide a global meaning and structure to their application.

Unlike integrative medicine, holistic medicine does have a philosophy behind it, namely that a human being is a whole organism of mind/body/spirit, and we can't separate out those elements when we look at health.

But holistic health is often put into practice without the defined scientific underpinnings of ultraprevention. Too frequently doctors who follow the holistic model are either out of date on current research, or don't make an effort to blend modern medicine into their practice. "What has worked over the centuries is good enough for us," they say, overlooking some of the most remarkable cures that any system, holistic or scientific, has come up with in just the last two or three years.

Too many doctors today follow no particular system at all. They simply do what they see as their basic job, which is to attack any illness a patient consults them about, and hope for the best.

Everyone can participate in ultraprevention. You don't have to visit Canyon Ranch. By understanding what you've read in Part I and are about to read in Part II, and by following the suggestions in Part III, you will possess everything you need to know to stay as healthy as possible.

But to give you a better idea of what we do here: We provide the most comprehensive total-immersion health program possible. We make sure our guests eat the best foods and engage in appropriate health-supporting activities, such as exercise programs and relaxation techniques like yoga, Tai Qi, meditation, and deep breathing. We also conduct extensive examinations to find out how we can better our patients' health—even those patients who aren't aware that anything is wrong with them.

During the exam we ask questions that are not usually asked in a medical interview. We ask about childhood and family history, about habits, about the chronology of any illness, about the conditions that preceded it, and what might have triggered it. We ask specifics about diet, food preferences, substance use, allergies and sensitivities, sleep patterns, stress levels, job satisfaction, daily schedules, important relationships, sex, digestive symptoms and patterns, brain function and mood, as well as making a head-to-toe review of all symptoms.

By the time we are finished, we have come up with a very different kind of story, one in which lifestyle and other details are essential to an understanding of the patient's condition. We consider that information and, if appropriate, we then conduct tests. If we suspect inflammation, we might look for various sources of inflammation, such as food allergies, or problems with digestive function, or disturbances of the gut immunity, or the presence of toxic substances, any or all of which can be remedied to reduce the inflammatory burden.

We would then send the patient to a nutritionist to learn how foods such as turmeric, cumin, rosemary, and ginger can impact the inflammatory response. We may recommend the patient reduce his or her inflammatory foods, such as animal proteins. We may increase his or her anti-inflammatory fats, such as omega-3 fatty acids, prescribing sardines and other fish.

We also perform a series of tests to look at biomarkers, which are indicators of health and wellness that we can measure and track over time to give us an idea of our patients' ongoing health, and which areas need particular attention. Some examples of biomarkers include body mass index and lean body mass, waist-to-hip ratio, acuity of vision and hearing, lung capacity and function, bone density, oxygen consumption (VO2 max), metabolic rate, blood pressure during exercise, memory and reaction time.

When most physicians test, they look for normal and abnormal levels. We do, too, but take it a step further—we look at the normal, the abnormal, and we look at the ideal, which is a much different concept. We would like to see values not just in the normal range, but in the ideal, or optimal range.

Is it okay if your thyroid function is on the borderline between normal and abnormal? What if your blood sugar is 126 instead of 127 (which is considered the cutoff level for diabetes)? Yes, you're not diabetic, but is that level okay? No, it's not.

Take the case of Fred, a lawyer who came to see us two months ago when his wife gave him a weekend at Canyon Ranch as an anniversary present. At three hundred pounds, Fred wasn't in good shape. He never exercised and he was coping with a host of serious health-related issues: high blood pressure, high cholesterol, and diabetes.

His doctor, who had reached these diagnoses following a routine examination, placed Fred on diabetic medication, as well as two medications for high blood pressure and two more for high cholesterol. He didn't consider any other treatments because, as he told Fred, the drugs were sufficient.

But these medications were causing various side effects: Fred was easily fatigued, badly constipated, and had no sex drive. Most depressing, Fred's doctor had told him that these conditions were basically irreversible.

Every time Fred returned to his doctor, his blood sugar tested higher. So the doctor increased Fred's dosages, creating a vicious cycle: The medication to treat his high blood pressure was making Fred's diabetes worse; to remedy the situation, he had to take more medication for his diabetes.

There are two types of diabetes. Juvenile-onset, or Type 1, diabetes (the type usually contracted when young), indicates a damaged pancreas that has stopped making insulin. Insulin is required to maintain a normal blood sugar level, so diabetic children typically need regular insulin injections or they become ill. However, in the adult form of diabetes (adult-onset, or Type 2), the reverse is usually true: Rather than not making enough insulin, the pancreas produces too much, and the body becomes progressively immune, or resistant to, its effects, just as the body develops some tolerance to anything it has to deal with regularly, from alcohol to caffeine. Because of this resistance, it has always been thought that Type 2 diabetics need still more insulin.

Most of the oral medications prescribed for diabetes work by making the pancreas manufacture more insulin. With these insulin-promoting medications, which were developed years ago when Western medicine thought more insulin was the only solution to diabetes, the dose must be gradually increased until most patients have to take insulin injections to get a sufficient dosage.

Back to Fred. We told him he could reverse his diabetes, his high blood pressure, and his cholesterol level. And that he didn't need drugs to do it.

We immediately started him on a program to lose weight as well as to control his diabetes and his high cholesterol. The right approaches to these issues would resolve his high blood pressure as well.

Because he had diabetes, Fred had been told he should be on a low-fat diet. So the man was stuffing himself with white pasta, white potatoes, white bread, and white rice, thinking all the while that this would improve his cholesterol levels. Instead they got worse and worse.

As we have seen, reducing the amount of fat in the diet is not the solution. The solution is controlling the fat levels in the blood. To do that, you must restrict foods that are rapidly turned into sugar in the body, as these white carbohydrates are; the carbohydrates then turn into fat in the form of triglycerides, and lower HDL, the good cholesterol.

We told Fred to increase his intake of fiber by eating legumes and other vegetables, and to add essential fats critical for insulin function and general health through consuming avocados, nuts, olive oil, seeds, and fish. Soon enough, although he was eating more fat, Fred was losing weight—a couple of pounds a week. Best of all, he liked his new diet.

But there was no way, he said, he could become an athlete. "No need," we said. "Just walk." So Fred started a two-mile-a-day walking program, improving his muscle mass and burning calories in a manner he enjoyed. It had never occurred to him that walking was considered exercise.

We also prescribed a specific supplement plan to remedy his previously unhealthy lifestyle; his unhappy cycle of medications, illness, and then more medications had led to a number of nutritional imbalances. So Fred's program included daily supplements of needed nutrients as we monitored his results.

When we next saw Fred, he was ecstatic. He had lost seventy-five pounds, his body had improved its sensitivity to insulin, his blood sugar had dropped, and his pancreas, not surprisingly, was producing less insulin. His cholesterol had also dropped down to a reasonable level and his blood pressure, too, was much lower. Best of all, he was no longer diabetic. As a result, he cut back on all his medications. He told his wife his stay at Canyon Ranch was the best anniversary present of his life.

No matter how old you are, you are the right age to start ultraprevention.

Question: How many twenty-year-olds have doctors and see them regularly? Few, except pregnant women who need an OB/GYN. How many thirty-year-olds? Not that many more. How many forty-year-olds? They're starting to have, and regularly see, doctors. How many fifty-year-olds? Most of them. That's because doctors can't offer much to someone who's in good health at age twenty-five. Because until a disease comes along, there's not much doctors can do—there's nothing to diagnose. But when you're fifty, suddenly your doctor has plenty to say to you—probably more than you'd like.

On the other hand, ultraprevention applies to people of any age. In fact, the younger you start, the better, because that is when you can identify those imbalances that need to be addressed, so that your life will be as healthy as possible. It's like an individual retirement account. The sooner you open a retirement account, the healthier your retirement will be, financially. It's the same with ultraprevention: The sooner you start working on it, the healthier your retirement will be, physically.

We recently saw a woman named Mona who told the sad tale of her daughter Angela, a twelve-year-old with a weight problem so out of control that Mona couldn't find any clothes to fit her. Mona had to buy Angela adult women's dresses that, too long, needed alterations and never truly looked good on her.

We asked if Angela had any health issues. "She does have quite a sweet tooth," her mother admitted. When we asked if this might be related to any family history, Mona said that Angela's father had been diabetic; she wondered if there was a connection.

When Mona brought Angela to her own doctor, he found that Angela's cholesterol was too high and he recommended a low-fat diet. Even so, Angela didn't lose weight.

Mona knew nothing about Angela's insulin, glucose, triglycerides, and HDL and LDL levels, so we decided to check those. The results were no surprise to us, but they were eye-opening to Mona.

Angela's triglyceride level was 285 (remember, this should be less than 100). Her glucose (or blood sugar) was 115, near the top of the normal range of 75 to 120. (The normal range for blood sugar may be 75 to 120, but the ideal range is 75 to 90.) Angela's total cholesterol was indeed high, at 225, but the level of HDL, or good cholesterol, was low, and her LDL level was quite high.

Worst, Angela's insulin level was 77, or over three times the norm. Furthermore, Angela's level of C-reactive protein (a protein that rises in the bloodstream in response to inflammation) was elevated at 4.0 (the ideal is less than 0.7), indicating inflammation in her bloodstream. We also found evidence of oxidative stress.

We told Mona that Angela had not just a weight problem, but that she suffered from what we call metabolic obesity caused by insulin resistance. Even though she was only twelve years old, Angela had the risk profile of a sixty-year-old with borderline diabetes.

Angela seemed to have inherited this tendency from her father, but the problem had been magnified and accentuated by her diet. Because her doctor only went as far as a diagnosis of high cholesterol and obesity, he failed to check her levels of insulin, the degree of inflammation, and the balance of good and bad cholesterol and triglycerides.

Instead of a low-fat diet, which aggravates the vicious cycle of insulin resistance, Angela was crying out for a completely different approach to eating. Such a diet included higher amounts of healthy fat, an increase in fiber and lean protein, and a sharp reduction in sugar, refined grains, and carbohydrates.

If not treated properly, Angela's condition would have become steadily worse until she eventually came down with diabetes, hypertension, and cardiovascular disease. In all likelihood she would also have suffered from irregular menstrual cycles, recurring ovarian cysts, and abnormal hair growth—all a result of the insulin resistance.

To keep this from taking place, we started Angela on an ultraprevention program, changing her diet, adding crucial supplements, and having her walk every morning with her mom. Not surprisingly, she steadily lost weight, while her blood pressure came down to 110/70 and her cholesterol dropped to 130—all in just six weeks.

When Mona told her doctor that the key to Angela's improving health had been to increase her fat intake, along with giving her the supplements, he told her outright that she had to be wrong. Instead he attributed the success to the new walking program, which was indeed a key component. But the doctor simply couldn't believe that added fat and vitamins could be so crucial.

We feel there are enormous advantages in store for anyone who comes on board the ultraprevention system. What more could you ask for than to feel as good as you possibly can? This should be every human's right: to achieve his or her best possible health.

But the benefits of ultraprevention go beyond the individual. One of our major goals is one that we think all societies should aspire to: the compression of morbidity. This means whole populations enjoying a long, healthy existence that ends with a short, fatal illness (or perhaps you die without any illness at all).

Instead of picking up diseases, dwindling, and losing function from age sixty on, people should ideally maintain their level of functioning until their eighties or even later, at which point the morbidity would occur, briskly ending good health and life at once.

The quality of our lives would be immeasurably improved by maintaining our independence, vitality, and productivity throughout our entire existence. We would also save immense amounts of time and money if we could keep ourselves vital and productive members of society during those otherwise often nonfunctional years. When we die young, we often pass through a long, expensive, and painful process of dying; when we die older, we are more likely to die quickly, cheaply, and painlessly.

The theory of compressed morbidity was first developed twenty years ago by Dr. James Fries, professor of medicine at Stanford University. Fries postulated that if people remained at their normal body weight, exercised vigorously, and didn't smoke, they would not only live longer, but would become sick only as they edged toward death.

The reaction? Like Dr. Kilmer McCully, who pointed out the importance of homocysteine levels, Fries was laughed out of the halls of the academic and the scientific research communities; the latter felt that if implemented, Fries's ideas would simply create a population of older, sicker people. So Fries spent decades proving his theory. Just five years ago, he published results in the *New England Journal of Medicine* (April 9, 1998) confirming that people who followed his rules regarding exercise, body weight, and cigarettes indeed lived longer, healthier lives than those who didn't.

Because ultraprevention is more than a smart and realistic system of health for an individual, we believe it can create a healthy world, too. Why? Because if people were healthy at the level that ultraprevention can provide, they would be freed from all the effort and details currently required to attend to personal health.

First of all, imagine if all those hundreds of billions of dollars spent on health care dwindled to a few billion. Finally, we could have an enduring budget surplus. And if we spent that money wisely, imagine the possible outcomes: We could develop cleaner sources of energy, feed the world's hungry, help prevent wars, or develop other programs that have been inhibited by lack of money.

And think about the equivalent increase in time. If we weren't sick, disabled, or unable to work, we could all be more productive. Think about how much more time we would have for other satisfying endeavors, such as the arts, philanthropy, or creative ventures.

We also believe that when people are in good health, they begin to reach out into their community to help those less fortunate.

As Heterophiles, the father of anatomy (and physician to Alexander the Great), wrote in 300 B.C.: "When health is absent, wisdom cannot reveal itself; art cannot become manifest; strength cannot be exerted; wealth is useless, and reason is powerless."

Thus we see health intervention as not just a way of healing an individual, but—applied most idealistically—as a way to help heal the planet.

## THE FIVE FORCES OF ILLNESS

As many Western doctors and scientists have realized over the last few years, the human body has an innate capacity to maintain its own health through complicated mechanisms our species has developed over centuries of evolution.

Nonetheless, at times, illness happens. As we have often said (and expect to say again and again for the rest of our careers), it's not always a disease that causes illness. Illness results when one or more of the five forces take hold. Some of these may sound familiar, such as malnutrition, but we don't mean the term in the way you probably think.

When we talk about these five forces with our patients, we refer to them metaphorically as sludge (malnutrition), burnout (impaired metabolism), heat (inflammation), waste (impaired detoxification), and rust (oxidative stress). The presence of these forces begins a chain of events that can set off a course of bad health in anyone, for the duration of your lifetime, whether you're eighteen or ninety-eight.

Let's now look at each one individually.

# FORCE 1: MALNUTRITION, OR SLUDGE

For most people, the word *malnutrition* conjures up images of starving children with swollen bellies and the skeletal appearance of skin stretched over bones. This severe form of malnutrition, or protein-calorie malnutrition, is seldom seen in the United States.

Yet over 80 percent of Americans are malnourished, even by the government's own assessments. It is a different kind of malnutrition, one that we call overconsumptive undernutrition.

What it means is that Americans are taking in too many calories yet too few nutrients. According to the USDA, 80 percent of Americans are not getting even the RDA of one or more of the essential vitamins, minerals, or other nutrients. And 91 percent are not eating the government's recommendation of *five* servings of fruits and vegetables a day. Yet we recommend eight to ten servings, not five!

The main areas of malnutrition among Americans include:

- Essential fatty acids
- Essential minerals:
  - Magnesium
  - Zinc
  - Calcium
  - Selenium
- Folic acid and the B-complex vitamins, which help to reduce homocysteine
  - Antioxidants

To complicate matters even further, it isn't always enough to simply eat the right kinds of food and take the right vitamins. In order for our bodies to be able to use the nutrients in our food, we must also have normally functioning *digestion* and *absorption* of the food we eat.

Most of us think that if our diets include ample amounts of lean meats, fruits, cereals, and vegetables, and we avoid fatty items like fudge cakes and deep-fried snacks, we don't have to consider the possibility of malnutrition.

Sorry—not so. Although diet is indeed an important factor in nutrition, it isn't the only one. How your body processes food is as important as the food itself. If your twin systems of digestion and absorption are not working well, you won't be healthy, no matter how healthful your diet. You will suffer—believe it or not—from malnutrition.

Digestion isn't as simple as people think. Most of us believe that if we eat something, we digest it—end of story. But it's not a given that good digestion always happens. In fact, bad digestion is so common it's given birth to a huge industry: all the antacids and the prescription-strength medications used to alleviate a world of upset stomachs.

When digestion works well, you take in the energy of the sun stored in food, and the minerals and vitamins that food has absorbed from the soil, and all the other wonderful and important plant molecules (phytonutrients) whose workings we haven't yet unraveled but which seem to have specific therapeutic effects in the human body.

These substances include isoflavones; genistein and daidzein, found in foods such as soy, whole grains, or beans; carotenoids, including beta-carotenes; and lutein and lycopene, found in tomatoes, yellow and orange fruits, and vegetables, and which have powerful anticancer properties.

Then these items are broken down into their component parts through a series of digestive steps that begin with chewing, followed by the enzymatic action of saliva, and then the mechanical churning in the stomach. This is followed by the release of acid (produced by the stomach) and digestive enzymes (from the stomach, pancreas, and liver). Further breakdown of food and fibers is performed by helpful bacteria that inhabit the intestinal tract.

Basically, digestion is what your stomach and your gastrointestinal tract do for a living: They break down all the food you eat—the fats, the carbohydrates, the proteins.

Protein is broken down to its component amino acids, which are the building blocks of protein. Carbohydrates are broken down into sugars, which are the building blocks of carbohydrates. Fats, too, are broken down into their own building blocks: fatty acids.

All of these complex foods must be reduced back to their simple building blocks in order to be absorbed and assimilated by our cells. If they're not broken down well, problems arise.

Here's the idea: Suppose someone injects beef directly into your bloodstream. You will develop a horrible allergic reaction and perhaps even die—humans are so different from cows that your immune system would immediately freak out. But if you first broke that cow protein down into its component amino acids, you could inject all the cow you wished into the bloodstream, and no reaction would result. The body knows what to do with amino acids. So the difference between life and death is the proper breakdown of foods.

How does digestion cause this breakdown?

There are three types of digestive juices. One is hydrochloric acid (made by the stomach). Then there are enzymes (made by the stomach and pancreas). The last is bile (made by the liver). So if the stomach, the pancreas, and the liver aren't doing their jobs properly, improper digestion results.

When digestion isn't working well, the most common culprit is a lack of stomach acid. A number of conditions can reduce the output of these digestive juices.

A primary factor is aging, which reduces the stomach's ability to produce acid. Another is damage to the stomach lining caused by an infection—for instance, the bacteria *Helicobacter* can injure this lining and, if allowed to continue, can severely impair the stomach's ability to produce acid. There's also a condition known as pernicious anemia, in which the stomach loses its ability to create acid because of a loss of certain stomach cells called the parietal cells (which release the acid). One result is that, without stomach acid, your body can't absorb minerals or vitamin $B_{12}$ (making you anemic—vitamin $B_{12}$ is essential for the proper production of red blood cells by the bone marrow).

Another potential problem: You may not be producing adequate amounts of digestive enzymes to break down food properly. Perhaps you are ingesting foods or medicines that impair digestion, such as antacids. Antacids may relieve some symptoms of indigestion, yet they also impair normal function. Stomach acid is required to activate the enzymes made by the stomach and pancreas to aid in the digestion process; without it, these enzymes cannot do their job.

Or, if you don't have the right bacteria in your gut, your body can't produce some of the key vitamins, like biotin, or vitamin K, which is actually manufactured by certain gut bacteria. (Recently vitamin K deficiency was found to be as big a risk factor for heart attack as smoking!)

Problems in the pancreas also can wreak havoc on digestion. The pancreas has two functions. One is digestive, the other hormonal (to control your blood sugar by making insulin). Its digestive function is to produce enzymes that break down fats, proteins, and carbohydrates. Whenever you eat, the pancreas releases its enzymes into the intestines, where they help digest food.

Many conditions and unhealthy practices can affect the pancreas and its ability to manufacture these juices, most commonly consumption of alcohol. Excessive alcohol consumption is a common cause of pancreatitis, or inflammation of the pancreas. Pancreatitis produces enough scarring and damage to impair the pancreas's digestive function. Other causes of pancreatitis include gallstones, viruses (primarily the mumps virus), and many medications.

Other problems may include an obstruction in the flow of pancreatic juices—this commonly happens due to the presence of a stone, like a gallstone that lodges in the pancreas's drainage area, blocking it. This forces the juices to back up into the pancreas; the pancreas ends up more or less digesting itself. As with the stomach, trouble also comes in the form of autoimmune diseases, in which the body makes an antibody that attacks the pancreas and stops the flow of its juices. A congenital ailment, such as cystic fibrosis, a disease that causes pancreatic insufficiency, may also affect pancreatic function. But it isn't necessary to have a serious condition for your pancreas to pump out less than the proper amounts and proportions of digestive juices your body requires every day.

On to the liver, which has multiple functions. One of these is the manufacture of bile, an emulsifier for fat; if not emulsified, fat cannot be absorbed into the bloodstream. Bile is manufactured in the liver and stored in the gallbladder. When you eat, the gallbladder squeezes and releases the bile into the duodenum (the first segment of the intestinal tract) and the intestine.

Problems that block this process include, of course, having your gallbladder removed, or having a damaged liver (through hepatitis, alcohol consumption, a number of drugs and toxins, gallstones, hormone imbalances, or autoimmune diseases). And there is a genetic disposition to bad bile—many families are prone to getting gallstones.

Healthy liver functioning is also important and necessary for proper digestion of food.

Recently we saw Wendy, a young woman who thought she was taking all the right vitamins and eating the right foods. But when we completed our tests, we found that she had an overgrowth of bad bacteria and an inadequate amount of good bacteria in her gut.

Wendy also lacked the proper enzyme function and enough stomach acids—all of which meant she wasn't breaking down her food properly. She was actually malnourished, even though she was eating a healthful diet and taking all the correct supplements.

What could have caused this? In Wendy's case, it turned out to be years of taking antibiotics, which her dermatologist had prescribed to her for a skin condition.

But this syndrome can also result from years of stress, or from not having enough good bacteria in the diet, or from taking drugs that change the balance in the gut, or from aging, which changes the stomach's level of acidity—over time, you can't produce as much stomach acid as a young person, and this creates an imbalanced ecology in your gut.

While *digestion* means breaking food down into components, *absorption* means getting it from the gut into the bloodstream. But that process doesn't always work properly, either; even though you might be digesting well, you could still suffer from malabsorption. Without good absorption, your system won't profit from whatever wonderful things you are putting into it.

Let's say that your gallbladder has been removed. Because your bile is not being stored up in the gallbladder, when you eat a fatty meal, there is not enough bile to emulsify your fats. Those fats are now undigested, and enter the intestine, where they can't be absorbed well because the large fat molecules haven't been broken down into smaller pieces. The fat, never absorbed, exits your body with the stool.

When you examine a stool you should not find any carbohydrates, fats, or proteins. Our bodies rely on these food components for nutrition, so it would be foolish to lose them in the stool—and our bodies seldom want to act foolishly. So we should see only those things that our bodies can't use for energy—fiber and waste products that we can't process. Anytime we find sugar, or fat, or protein in the stool, we know we are dealing with a patient who is suffering from malabsorption.

Or let's say the lining of the bowel is damaged, as in colitis or gastroenteritis. If you've ever had the latter, you know that painful feeling when, after you've eaten, the food seems to go right through your system. That's because, due to inflammation, you can't absorb the food in the colon or the intestines. You see this condition in HIV patients; they come down with chronic diarrhea that leads to malabsorption, and then they start wasting away—they are malnourished because they can't absorb the food they are eating.

A similar process occurs artificially when people eat the synthetic fat known as Olestra, a new product on the supermarket shelves that was actually designed to cause malabsorption. Because Olestra can't be absorbed from the gut, the "fat" in the food ends up going right through the body, meaning it doesn't add any extra pounds, but it can cause diarrhea. Worse, in the process of malabsorbing the fat, the body also doesn't absorb important fat-soluble nutrients such as vitamins A, D, E, and K. This can lead to serious complications such as heart attacks, bleeding, osteoporosis, and the inability to quench free radicals, leading to oxidative damage.

The most common cause of malabsorption is a commonly missed condition known as celiac disease. As reported recently in the *New England Journal of Medicine* (January 17, 2002), an increasing awareness of this condition among physicians has made them realize that what was once thought to be a rare disorder is quite common—it affects as many as one out of every 120 people in the United States and Europe.

Celiac disease is caused by an allergy to gluten, a protein found in wheat and wheat-containing foods, as well as in several other common grains such as rye, barley, and oats. The disease causes malabsorption by damaging the lining of the small intestine, damage caused by the immune system as it creates an inflammatory reaction to the gluten protein in individuals who have become allergic to it. The disorder also causes hypoglycemia (low blood sugar), diarrhea, skin rashes, canker sores in the mouth, slowing of growth in children, and autoimmune diseases including diabetes and thyroid disease.

Successful treatment of celiac disease requires elimination of gluten from the diet; this includes all wheat, rye, and barley products, as well as any other foods or medications containing gluten (of which there are many), and even beers and ales, which are made from wheat. When gluten is properly eliminated from the diet, the conditions arising from celiac disease, including the malabsorption, resolve.

Jim is a thirty-eight-year-old salesman with a history of diarrhea for as long as he can remember. Over the years he had seen his doctor many times and had been referred to countless gastroenterologists, but none of them ever diagnosed a problem; instead, they said his diarrhea wasn't serious and prescribed Lomotil, an antimotility drug that slows down the normal movement of the bowel. Unfortunately, this did not help much and Jim simply lived with his chronic diarrhea, thinking that it was somehow normal for him.

When we first saw Jim and asked him our long series of questions, the problem quickly became clear. He complained of canker sores in his mouth and an intermittent skin rash on his chest, and he noted that whenever he drank beer, he sneezed. He was also fairly short, while his parents were both tall (celiac disease causes short stature if it's present during a child's growth years).

That was enough for us. Blood tests confirmed celiac disease—Jim had a high level of antibodies to gluten. He soon began a gluten-free diet. Within two weeks, his diarrhea had disappeared, along with his other symptoms. (Okay, he didn't grow any taller, but he was no longer bothered by the symptoms of celiac.)

Remember: Our immune system fights off any potentially toxic invaders trying to get into our system, such as bacteria, germs, microbes, and parasites, and it's always on surveillance, looking for something it needs to attack.

A foreign object can get into our system via one of four routes: through the skin, the respiratory tract (via the nose or lungs), sexual contact, or the gastrointestinal tract. The latter presents the biggest risk, because the surface area of the gastrointestinal tract is literally the size of a tennis court. A border this size requires a great deal of surveillance; otherwise the many germs in the gastrointestinal tract can cross the intestinal lining and enter the bloodstream, causing an immediate and profound response by the immune system.

Our immune system has to be very smart about killing and attacking bacteria. It doesn't want to attack its own body, so it has to be able to recognize what's "you" and what's "not you." The way it does that is by identifying which proteins are yours and which are foreign.

Any protein that is not recognized as yours is considered a potential invader and attacked. So if you eat a food or protein and don't digest it completely—if you don't break that protein down into the component building blocks—you'll have an immune reaction. And that can be detrimental, since you don't want to mount an immune reaction to every food you eat. When this reaction occurs, you can get inflammatory bowel disease, arthritis, acne, eczema, psoriasis, hives, liver problems, and so on.

And if you were to eat that protein again—let's say it's milk—and it wasn't completely digested, but entered your bloodstream in a nondigested or partially digested form—your immune system would make an antibody against milk, thinking that it is a foreign protein. Then the next time you drank milk, your immune system would be activated, up and ready to fight this alien milk (thinking it is a foreign protein, a potential invader), and that reaction would in turn make you feel sick.

Unfortunately, these antibodies can linger for up to several weeks in our bloodstream, long after the food that activated them is gone, and thus they can sometimes miss their target and attack other parts of the body, including the thyroid, the pancreas, the joints, or the cells themselves. So incomplete digestion can lead to allergies as well as to autoimmune diseases, which arise when our antibodies are actually attacking our own tissues.

The easiest test for this kind of malnutrition is simply to examine the stool to see if fats, carbohydrates, or proteins are present. If they are, either the digestion or absorption process has gone awry. A blood test can also be revealing; if you have low levels of building blocks like amino acids, then you're probably not absorbing or digesting well. Symptoms are another clue—if you suffer from digestive problems like constant diarrhea, or abdominal pain, or constipation, you could be suffering malnutrition.

If you can locate such a problem, you can also find a solution. For example, if weak stomach acid is an issue, we recommend stomach acid supplements. If there's an irritation in the lining of the intestine that's blocking absorption, then treatment is directed at healing this lining in order to restore normal functioning. If the culprit is poor gallbladder function caused by a medication or a poor diet, then we can address those specific causes as well.

One very simple way to improve gallbladder function is to increase the proportion of healthy fat in the diet. For years doctors have known that low-fat diets lead to sluggish gallbladder function, stagnation of the bile, and gallstones. (So have many lawyers, who have repeatedly brought suits against many of the well-known national weight-loss programs.) The obvious solution to insufficient healthy fat in the diet is to eat more of it.

A problem with the pancreas is harder to remedy, because this organ is complex but delicate. There are, however, pancreatic enzymes that can be added to a diet—people with cystic fibrosis take them, because cystic fibrosis causes pancreatic insufficiency.

Good nutrition means delivering all of the necessary nutrients in the correct proportions to the cells in our bodies that need them. Achieving this goal is much more complicated than simply eating the right foods. If there are problems with digestion, absorption, or delivery of these nutrients, your cells can't function properly and malnutrition, or sludge, occurs. This sludge interferes with our cells' ability to function optimally, and is thus a sign of the beginnings of illness.

# FORCE 2: IMPAIRED METABOLISM, OR BURNOUT

Whenever we feel what is generally called burnout, we endure a loss of energy. Most of us are all too aware of this unhappy state when we feel we simply don't have enough get-up-and-go; indeed, we'd rather just lie-down-and-stop.

But burnout isn't just a loss of energy on that familiar level that we all feel now and then. It applies all the way down to the cellular level.

Normally, your cells perform necessary daily functions: Your muscle cells contract, your liver cells detoxify, your brain cells fire the chemical impulses we call thought. To perform these functions they need energy.

Burnout means the loss of that cellular energy. It indicates that your metabolism isn't working well. This also implies that you're suffering from still another food-related problem, because *metabolism* is the term used to describe the creation of usable energy for all bodily functions from food. In other words, it is the process of converting food into energy. An impaired metabolism can lead to countless dysfunctions, from insulin resistance to the loss of muscle power, from a lack of overall energy to Alzheimer's disease.

When our metabolism is functioning properly, it works like this: When we eat, first we digest, then we absorb (or properly channel the nutrients into cells), and finally we burn that food to produce energy. In the process we create a high-energy fuel, our body's gasoline: adenosine triphosphate, or ATP.

ATP is an excellent source of energy for our bodies because it is portable; within the cell, ATP can be transported to wherever it's needed. The energy is stored within the ATP molecule as a high-energy chemical bond, sort of like a spring-loaded device. Just unhook the spring and—boom!—you release energy.

This bond can be unhooked by a readily available enzyme in each of our cells. When those bonds are broken, and the energy is released, that energy is used by the brain to think, by the heart to beat, and as far as science now knows, by every cell in your body to perform its particular function.

Your body makes two thirds of its own weight each day in ATP; the average 150-pound human makes up to a hundred pounds of ATP every twenty-four hours!

In its natural state, the body, which is programmed to work well, efficiently converts food into energy. But the conditions under which the body was programmed were those of our ancestors. For prehistoric humans, food was not a plentiful thing, but an intermittent and much welcomed acquisition.

Over the eons, our bodies learned to adapt so that when we did find food, we could eat all of it at once; our body then stored away the energy we didn't need immediately in the form of fat. Fat is a very high-energy but low-weight type of fuel; it's easy to carry around because it weighs half as much as protein or starch but provides the equivalent amount of energy.

The practice of eating only when we could find food has changed dramatically as humankind has surrounded itself with many modern conveniences, not the least of which is the refrigerator. Our bodies are not quite as smart as they used to be. They don't have to be.

The raw materials for your metabolism come from your diet, or the fuel that you put into your body that makes your cells function. If you put junk in, you get junk out. In other words, many things can go wrong when you eat poorly.

For example, when you eat hydrogenated fat (those synthetic fats created in the laboratory by chemically altering naturally occurring fats), your body is tricked into thinking it is real food because hydrogenated fats taste like fat, even though the body can't make use of them as with normal dietary fats.

However, we lack the necessary enzymes to process these synthetic fats, and because they can't be processed properly, they cause problems. The body's cells incorporate the hydrogenated fats into the cell membranes, where they interfere with normal cellular function, gumming up the works by making the cell membranes stiffer and less fluid.

We've talked about how important it is that our cell membranes remain fluid, smooth, and responsive. Cell membranes—all 100 trillion of them—must be fluid to do their job well.

But when a twisted fatty-acid molecule, such as a trans fat, is incorporated into the cell membrane lining, it puts a kink in that membrane, making it less fluid, and keeping it from communicating well with its neighbors.

That membrane is the interface between all the cells; it controls how things enter and leave the cells, how the cells "talk" to one another, how they do their job at keeping out invaders and absorbing nutrients. Thus the function of the cell will be fundamentally altered, no matter what its function is, if these stiff fats are incorporated into the cell membrane.

Most people think about their health on a large-scale basis. Is the whole system (you) feeling well? As the above example hints, metabolism actually occurs on a cellular level. It's not something that happens in your stomach, or in your intestinal tract. Metabolism happens inside the cells all over your body. And health problems begin on the cellular level, where they can smolder for years before symptoms or illness become manifest.

When working with our patients on the issue of metabolism, we focus on certain areas.

One of these is insulin. We've talked about insulin before, but it's so important that we probably can't bring it up enough.

A hormone manufactured by the pancreas, insulin's main function is to regulate the level of sugar (or glucose) in the bloodstream. This is a critical function, because glucose is the main fuel for all of our energy needs (ATP is made from glucose, so in a sense, ATP is like gasoline, glucose like crude oil).

Our brain runs exclusively on glucose; when blood sugar begins to drop, you will first feel irritable, then confused, and eventually comatose. So it's critical for our bodies to regulate and control the bloodstream's glucose level.

When you eat a meal, food is digested in the stomach and the intestinal tract, and then is absorbed into the bloodstream. Once this digested food enters the bloodstream, our pancreas releases a carefully metered amount of insulin.

The effect of this insulin is to move that food from the bloodstream into the cells, where the food can be metabolized—that is, where the food can be transformed into usable energy for our bodily functions.

If insulin is not functioning properly, digested food in the bloodstream is unable to enter the cells to provide energy, and metabolism is stalled. The blood becomes clogged with excessive amounts of food, including fats, cholesterol, sugar, and amino acids (the building blocks of protein). These sources of energy remain in the bloodstream and can't enter the cells, which, now starved for energy, start to malfunction.

This condition is known as insulin resistance; it occurs when the body loses its responsiveness to insulin and our cells are unable to derive energy from the food we eat. Even though we may have eaten an ample amount, our cells cry out for more food, which is translated by the brain into hunger. Despite having eaten plenty, we find ourselves tired and hungry again. Our brain then tells us to find a quick source of high energy, namely sugar, the most rapidly available source of energy.

When insulin works properly, it causes little pores found on the muscle cells to absorb all the food coming through the blood-stream—it's as though the insulin were opening a gate to let food inside. When you are insulin resistant, however, that gate becomes jammed, so you'll need more force to open it. To muster this kind of force, the body has to produce more and more insulin, so the insulin level goes up and up.

Think of what happens when you drink too much—the more you drink, the more tolerant you become of alcohol. The same is true of insulin. If you develop insulin resistance, you get hungrier and crave more sugar. The more sugar you eat, the more insulin is released by your pancreas. The more insulin released, the more tolerant, or resistant, your cells become to its effects. The gate remains stuck. This leads to a vicious cycle that produces higher and higher insulin levels, and more insulin resistance.

A drinker must stop drinking to lower tolerance levels. The same is true of insulin. In order to become sensitive and responsive to insulin again, you must reduce your production of insulin, by reducing your intake of the sugars and refined carbohydrates that trigger more and more insulin production.

Over the long term, insulin resistance leads to clogging of the arteries and heart disease, stroke, high blood pressure, and diabetes, and is also associated with hormonal cancers (such as breast or prostate cancer), as well as colon and pancreatic cancer. You are also at risk for dementia, because a higher level of insulin causes the brain to age more rapidly, as insulin resistance causes increased inflammation throughout the body.

Another metabolism-related issue is mitochondrial dysfunction.

We believe that individual cells have to function well for health to be optimal. Just as all the organs in your body are related, and taken together form an overall picture of health, every cell in your body, too, is part of a grand system, and all must be working in balance.

Mitochondria, a vital part of your cells' business, are subcellular organelles (tiny structures within the cells about the size of a bacterium) with their own unique membranes, or linings; this isolates them from the rest of the cell.

Mitochondria are so small that there can be thousands of them inside just one cell. They also have their own DNA, and are so similar to bacteria that some people think they may indeed be a kind of bacteria that began to exist with mammals in a symbiotic relationship many eons past.

Mitochondria are important because they are the body's energizers; it's inside the mitochondria where fuel (food) is actually burned to produce energy (ATP). In other words, they are tiny power plants.

Once food gets inside the cell, it enters the mitochondria, and these little organelles then take that fuel and turn it into energy, using oxygen. They do this by taking the sugar, fatty acids, or amino acids from what you eat, and the oxygen you breathe, and burn it, releasing energy, heat, and some waste.

Mitochondria burn fuel either well or badly, a little like a car that's fuel-efficient, or not. (If you have ever been behind a car that's not fuel-efficient, you can tell by the gassy smell.)

Mitochondria are present in proportion to the cell's energy needs: Those cells that need the most energy contain the greatest number of mitochondria. For example, each of your muscle cells has thousands and thousands of mitochondria in it. Fat cells may only have one hundred to two hundred mitochondria because, for the most part, they don't require much energy. The primary purpose of the fat cell is fat storage, whereas muscle cells are constantly being used.

The number of mitochondria determines the speed of metabolism—the more mitochondria, the faster the metabolism. (The amount of mitochondria varies not only from one organ to another, but also from one person to another. Part of this is genetic, but environmental factors can make a difference, including exercise: A more fit person would have better-functioning mitochondria and more per pound of body weight.)

An efficient metabolism is an excellent marker for health. After all, you want to use all of the calories you eat for energy rather than putting them into storage and getting fat. You can't do that if your mitochondria aren't functioning well. If they are sluggish or damaged, or you don't have enough of them, your metabolism won't be efficient, and your energy level will suffer. And if you don't have enough energy, then your health will start to fail.

Similarly, when disease strikes an organ, like the heart or the liver, it's the mitochondria that fail first. Then the heart or liver as an entire organ fails.

Mitochondria will fail for several reasons. Some of them are supposed to fail; science hasn't yet figured out why this is so, but it may have to do with a renewal process.

They also fail due to the lack of proper nutrients, or from oxidative damage. Because the process of burning calories to provide energy in the mitochondria requires oxygen, free radicals are produced as a by-product. These free radicals are also known as "reactive oxygen species," or ROS. Think of these ROS as the sparks that fly off a quickly burning fire. As our mitochondria burn fuel (food) to make energy, these sparks can burn and damage the mitochondria themselves. And as the mitochondria are damaged, they are no longer able to create energy for the cells, and the cells die.

Normally, our mitochondria have their own natural defenses against these sparks, a sort of built-in sprinkler system. This sprinkler system is the mitochondrial antioxidant system, composed of important antioxidants that can cool the heat and extinguish the sparks from the process of internal combustion inside the mitochondria. These antioxidants include important nutrients such as vitamin E, coenzyme Q10, alpha-lipoic acid, and superoxide dismutase.

Anything that interferes with this antioxidant system will allow for mitochondrial damage, which then leads to cell damage and death, as will deficiencies in these important antioxidants. High levels of oxidative stress (too strong a fire inside the mitochondria) will also overwhelm the antioxidant system and lead to damage.

Another common cause of mitochondrial damage is poisoning from heavy metals, petrochemicals, pesticides, and trans fats. One of the most frequently seen types of mitochondrial damage is from the heavy metal mercury. Mercury poisoning is much more common than most people think. We are exposed to mercury by eating large, predatory marine fish such as tuna, swordfish, mahi-mahi, halibut, and bluefish. Mercury exposure also results from silver (amalgam) dental fillings. Anyone who eats very large amounts of tuna and swordfish, and has a mouthful of amalgam fillings, risks possible mitochondrial damage.

When we examine disease and illness on a cellular level, we find mitochondrial damage or dysfunction occurring in almost every major type of illness, including Alzheimer's disease, hepatitis, heart disease, stroke, diabetes, and cancer. Protecting and caring properly for these vital little power plants, then, is a critical objective in promoting optimal health.

Another problem affecting metabolism is thyroid dysfunction.

The thyroid is a gland in the neck that produces two hormones that control a huge array of bodily functions: They set your body's temperature, control how often you have a bowel movement, determine the rate of your hair and nail growth, and they have a strong impact on your cholesterol levels, as well as your heart rate and your blood pressure.

If mitochondria are like power plants, then the thyroid gland is sort of like the gas pedal on your car. Too much thyroid hormone and everything speeds up. Too little thyroid, and everything slows down. Thus, if you have an excess of thyroid hormones, all your systems work more robustly: You need to go to the bathroom more often, your heart rate goes up, your nails grow faster, your body temperature is higher.

In other words, your metabolism is much higher. You can burn up more calories than most people, and you don't gain as much weight. This is called hyperthyroidism, and can lead to anxiety, sleeplessness, diarrhea, palpitations, and osteoporosis. But if your thyroid is sluggish, you're like a hibernating bear, who burns fewer calories than otherwise.

The thyroid can also be viewed as the body's thermostat. When thyroid level is low (or underactive), you become sluggish, your body temperature drops, and your appetite diminishes—yet you gain weight, your skin becomes oily and thick, your hair becomes coarse, your cholesterol starts to rise, your reflexes and your bowel function slow, you become constipated and depressed.

The thyroid can become underactive for a variety of reasons. The most common is an autoimmune disease in which the body makes an antibody that attacks the thyroid gland.

This seems to happen because, while trying to create an antibody against something else, an antibody is made that cross-reacts, or attacks the thyroid. What is it that the body was really targeting, and why did the bullet go astray and hit the thyroid gland? We don't know for sure, but this happens so much more often in women than in men that perhaps, during a pregnancy, the body makes an antibody against some part of the fetal cells, and the antibody attacks the mother's thyroid. It could also be triggered by an allergic reaction to food; toxins in air, water, and earth; an infection; malnutrition, such as a selenium deficiency; or low iodine levels. (Before salt was iodized, the presence of goiters, large, swollen thyroid glands protruding from the neck, was a common sign of iodine deficiency.)

There is a well-known association between celiac disease (wheat allergy) and autoimmune disease of the thyroid. Perhaps in the process of making antibodies to wheat, some antibodies to the thyroid are also created. Or perhaps someone with a digestive problem that leads to a wheat allergy might also be producing antibodies to several other foods, one of which may be attacking the thyroid. Although the cause is unclear, we can measure these antibodies in the bloodstream of someone who has thyroid dysfunction.

Because the thyroid gland is like the gas pedal of our metabolism, it's critically important to assess and promote healthy thyroid function in order to promote a healthy and intelligent metabolism.

The best way to measure metabolic fitness, we find, is to measure VO2 max. We feel the VO2 max indicator also correlates with overall health.

Remember, your metabolism burns food to produce energy. In doing that, it is using oxygen, as in any internal combustion machine. Food won't burn without the presence of oxygen.

VO2 max indicates the amount of oxygen your body uses to burn fuel (food). If your VO2 max is high, you are using a lot of oxygen to burn fuel. This means your metabolism is faster.

Think of two people unloading a cord of wood from a truck. One of them might unload that cord and burn 500 calories, the other 750. The latter's body is using more oxygen, is fitter, and is also more resistant to certain health problems.

There is a direct relationship between how much oxygen you breathe per minute and how many calories you can burn in that minute. If you can't breathe in enough air, your metabolic fuel efficiency will be low. And if little oxygen is getting to your mitochondria, they'll burn calories very slowly.

People don't think that poor fitness is a disease, but it is. Poor fitness is directly related to mortality. The lower your VO2 max and fitness level, the higher your risk of death.

The highest recorded male VO2 max measurement was 94 milliliters of oxygen per kilogram per minute. The highest recorded female measurement was 74 ml/kg/min. Cyclist Greg LeMond, three-time winner of the Tour de France, clocked a 92.5. Runner Steve Prefontaine, the former one-mile record holder, scored an 84. These unusually fit athletes burn fuel efficiently.

But most people aren't world-class athletes. When you exercise on a treadmill, or in step or aerobics class, or even if you're just walking quickly to the store, you can be burning between five and fifteen calories per minute. Healthwise, you would much rather be the person who is burning fifteen calories per minute than the person burning five calories.

The good news is that you can improve your VO2 max through certain forms of exercise, particularly interval training. Here you exercise through the usual target heart rate zone for aerobic exercise to a higher pulse rate closer to your maximum heart rate.

(Calculate your maximum heart rate by subtracting your age from 220—if you're fifty, your maximum heart rate is 170. Your target heart zone for aerobic exercise is between 70 and 85 percent of your maximum heart rate, in this case 119 to 145 beats per minute.)

During interval training, the goal is to exceed your target heart zone and get to a higher-intensity level of exercise, which usually begins at around 80 to 85 percent of your maximum heart rate. When your heart rate rises this high, you become anaerobic; that is, your muscles are requiring more oxygen than your heart and lungs are able to provide. This causes a buildup of lactic acid in the muscles, which is why you become so tired. Then you have to stop, breathe, and clear out all the lactic acid, which is released largely as carbon dioxide. Interval training is a strong stimulus for our muscles to make more mitochondria; because the heart and lungs can't provide any additional oxygen to the muscles, our muscles produce more mitochondria in order to extract more oxygen from the bloodstream.

In interval training, you work to the point of being anaerobic, then slow back down until you are in your aerobic range. Next you increase your effort until you go back to being anaerobic. Then you slow down again to the aerobic range.

For instance, during a thirty- to forty-five-minute workout, you would go as fast as you can for one minute, then slow down to 60 to 75 percent of your maximal heart rate for three minutes, and then go as fast as you can for two minutes, then go back to 60 to 75 percent of your maximal heart rate again. Back and forth, back and forth—in this manner you will improve your VO2 max.

The effect of this interval training is to increase your fitness, your VO2 max, your calories burned per minute, and your longevity as well as your mitochondrial function.

Note: A good VO2 max is often hereditary, which is why some people were born to be marathon runners; their bodies can soak up oxygen like crazy. Other people are born sprinters: They can run very fast for short distances, but they can't get anaerobic. They have power, but not endurance.

In short, if you don't burn oxygen efficiently, all that exercise you may be doing isn't helping you burn as many calories as you might think.

Efficient metabolism is one of the cornerstones of good health. When your body is efficiently burning all of the calories you eat, without storing up fat and without causing damage to your mitochondria, your long-term health outlook is positive. If your metabolism becomes sluggish or inefficient, as with insulin resistance, mitochondrial or thyroid dysfunction, or inefficient oxygen utilization, your health is headed for burnout problems, not to mention problems with your entire hormonal balance, including the balance of stress hormones, sex hormones, and growth hormone.

# FORCE 3: INFLAMMATION, OR HEAT

People probably spend more money trying to reduce their inflammation than on any other ailment. If you don't believe us, go look at the array of anti-inflammatory drugs in your local pharmacy: Advil, ibuprofen, Aleve, and aspirin, not to mention the myriad of prescription anti-inflammatories, including Celebrex and Vioxx, the recent pharmaceutical blockbusters.

There are five cardinal signs of inflammation in the body: redness, swelling, heat, pain, and loss of function.

Although most people think of inflammation simply as redness and swelling, it is actually the activation of the immune system due to the presence of some kind of intruder, such as an infection, allergen, or toxin.

Whenever you have any kind of inflammation, your body creates heat. This is because inflammation causes an increase in circulation as blood vessels dilate, triggering a rise in temperature.

Let's say you have inflammation—perhaps a reaction to poison ivy—on your skin, where the temperature is normally about 80 degrees. Your core temperature is much higher (98.6), so an increase in blood circulation at the site of inflammation causes warmth, because it brings heat from your body's core to your skin.

Any time your immune system is activated, inflammation results. It's as though the immune system had a volume knob. Normally this knob is turned low, as your immune system sits in a kind of surveillance mode, like a security camera, just looking around to see if something dangerous or alien is near. Anything that triggers the immune system, and turns that volume knob up to a noticeable level, will cause inflammation.

Often inflammation occurs in an area that can sense pain, like your knee, and you will usually experience some level of discomfort.

The problem is that even if inflammation is at a low level, it has the potential to cause serious illness—but you won't necessarily know about it because you can't feel it. It's like a smoldering fire. You may not be aware it's burning until the fire suddenly rages out of control.

These low levels of inflammation may only be detected by looking in the bloodstream, as we'll explain later. (And there's a difference between local inflammation, such as a bee sting, which doesn't cause inflammation throughout your body, and the systemic, generalized forms of inflammation we're now discussing.)

When your body's inflammation level is excessive, many serious conditions can result, such as Alzheimer's, arthritis, heart disease, diabetes, Parkinson's disease, or prostatitis. All of these ailments are related to the body's inability to control inflammation adequately.

Yet most common diseases involve some level of inflammation; in fact, we know many conditions are not truly dangerous unless they exist with inflammation.

Cholesterol, for instance, is a fat transported in the blood; it's a component of every cell in your body. At moderate levels cholesterol is a good thing—the body requires it, which is why the body manufactures it. All your sex hormones and adrenal hormones are made from cholesterol. The body doesn't tend to make too many things it doesn't need.

Cholesterol only causes a problem when it builds up in the wall of the arteries. And it can only get deposited in the wall of the artery if there is inflammation.

How that occurs is a complicated process. Think of inflammation as plaque formation, which is the starting point of the blockages that lead to heart attack and stroke. The cholesterol builds up under the surface of the artery wall, not unlike a pimple on your face. A pimple starts as a little white spot, then grows and becomes inflamed, red, and swollen. Finally it becomes infected and ruptures.

That same process occurs in the wall of the artery. The "pimple" (or plaque) grows and gets inflamed; it may become infected and then burst. When that pimple in the wall of the artery bursts, a blood clot forms at the location of the ruptured plaque. This small blood clot then blocks the circulation of blood into the artery. Depending on where the plaque was located, results could include heart attack, stroke, or damage to limbs or organs.

And only inflammation will make that pimple grow and burst.

Inflammation has many causes, including infections, allergies, lack of oxygen, free radicals and oxidative stress, exposure to toxins, insulin resistance, and obesity. It can result from everyday ailments such as bronchitis and sinus or bladder infections, as well as skin, dental, vaginal, or prostate infections.

Sometimes unusual or unsuspected infections trigger inflammation. These include Lyme disease and the bacterium that causes stomach ulcers, known as *Helicobacter pylori*. Infections with the bacteria called chlamydia have also been implicated as risk factors for heart disease and stroke. Specific testing may be required to identify these infections, since their symptoms are not always common ones such as fever or those associated with flu.

Allergens, both environmental and food-related, can also trigger inflammation. Grasses, pollens, and molds, as well as food items such as gluten (in wheat), cow's milk, and yeast products (baked goods, beer, and wine), are other common triggers.

Injury and trauma, too, can cause inflammation on a chronic basis. Whenever there is an injury, tissues are damaged, which causes the contents of the cells to leak out into the rest of the system, triggering inflammation. Injury also leads to lack of oxygen due to swelling and disruption of blood flow. The bigger the injury and its bruise, the more inflammation will result.

Poor circulation from any other cause also triggers inflammation, such as blood clots that shut off circulation (as in heart attack or stroke) or a strangulated hernia, in which the bowel pokes through a small hole in the groin and chokes circulation to that part of the bowel. The more tissue affected by poor circulation, the more inflammation is produced.

Also triggering inflammation are free radicals and oxidative stress, which can be caused by overeating, obesity, chronic infections, exposure to toxins, a diet poor in vegetables, or lack of fiber or essential fats—anything that depletes the body of antioxidants.

Other common sources of inflammation are toxins such as air or water pollution, pesticides, food additives, drugs, cosmetics, and household or workplace chemicals. Bacteria such as *E. coli* and anthrax cause illness by releasing toxins after they infect their host. Toxins can also be created by other microbes, bacteria, plants, or fungi, such as those produced by moldy peanuts.

Internal toxins are produced within the body, often by the digestive tract, where many microbes live. When these microbes fight among themselves, they release chemical toxins that we, their host, absorb. All these trigger inflammation.

And simply being overweight or having insulin resistance triggers inflammation. Often there is no reason for an elevated C-reactive protein level other than just carrying extra pounds, particularly around the middle of your body.

Although each of the sources of inflammation is different, one common end result occurs, and that is activation of the immune system. Whether we are dealing with an infection, an injury, oxidative stress, insulin resistance, or an allergy, the result is the same.

This immune activation is a hazard that spreads throughout your system, because the immune system travels through your bloodstream. So inflammation that starts in your big toe or in your teeth can travel and affect your heart, your liver, or your brain.

No wonder research shows that people with bad teeth are more prone to heart attacks, and that people with severe hepatitis (inflammation in the liver) can slip into a coma.

We feel that the most important aspect of inflammation is its relationship to the gut.

The gut is our largest interface with the outside world. It's the area where we most often come into contact with foreign substances, mainly (obviously) food and other things we may swallow, such as germs. People don't usually think of their intestinal tract as part of the outside world. But actually it is, since it communicates directly with the outside at both ends—the mouth and the anus. The lining of our gut acts as a filter between those things that are physically outside our cells (inside the "tube" of the gut) and inside our cells (inside "us").

There is a direct relationship between what happens in the digestive tract and what happens in the rest of the body regarding regulation of the immune response. Because the surface area of the intestinal tract is so large, our immune system contains a tremendous number of cells that are needed to control the security of the border between the rest of the body and the intestinal contents.

Think of the linings of your stomach and intestines as having a force field around them protecting you from outside invaders. When that force field breaks down for any number of reasons (such as stress, medications, infections, allergens, or inflammatory conditions such as colitis or ileitis), invaders can enter, and your immune system is activated.

When your immune cells recognize an invader, they spring into action, making antibodies, gobbling up invading germs, and calling in reinforcements (more immune cells) for backup support. A signal is sent out to the entire immune system that an invader is trying to gain access to the bloodstream, and this signal initiates the process of inflammation. This inflammation then leads to illnesses that are not necessarily felt in the gut, but originate there.

One way we measure the presence of inflammation in the system is through a blood test for what's known as C-reactive protein, a protein whose levels rise in the bloodstream in response to inflammation. Though other proteins react similarly, this particular one is so sensitive that it makes for an ideal marker that can be easily measured.

Usually when part of your body is inflamed, you know it. A shoulder may be sore due to bursitis; a stuffed-up nose causes pain due to sinusitis; a belly aches with appendicitis. But with the C-reactive protein test, we are able to look for mild forms of inflammation, the kinds you can't necessarily feel.

We believe everyone should take this test to look for signs of inflammation. The test won't tell you where the inflammation is coming from, but it can warn you that inflammation is present, and to be on the lookout for its cause.

Through experience we have found that if someone's C-reactive protein level is high, it often turns out to be a gut-related problem, because of bad food, an allergy, a parasite, an imbalance in bacteria, or some breakdown in the lining of the gut.

Recently we saw a man named Ray; during his routine checkup we discovered he had very high levels of C-reactive protein. We didn't know why, and so we ended up giving him a few more tests, including one for an unsuspected infection. It turned out he had two, both caused by unusual bacteria; both had been sexually transmitted. When he was treated with antibiotics, Ray's C-reactive protein level went back down.

★  ★  ★

Two of the most common and serious inflammation-related diseases are asthma and irritable bowel syndrome.

Few people think of asthma as inflammatory, but it is. When the bronchial tubes in the lungs become inflamed, they swell, causing shortness of breath and wheezing.

Asthma may be caused by common airborne allergens such as pollen, dust, dander, or mites. But it is not always related to something an individual has inhaled. Asthma can also be caused by food. People who are allergic to milk may well develop it. This is because when the immune system in the gut spots that milk, it says, "This is a foreign substance," and reacts by activating the immune response in the entire body, including the lungs; this results in the familiar symptoms of shortness of breath and wheezing.

Likewise, the ever-common irritable bowel syndrome is inflammation-related. The very presence of irritable bowel syndrome signals a damaged gut ecology. This is often due to an imbalance in the gut bacteria, perhaps because of improper digestion, which contributes to bloating and gas. Incomplete digestion of proteins leads to allergies, which then increase inflammation, not just in the gut but all over the body, particularly in the lungs.

*The Lancet* recently published (April 7, 2001) the results of a study in which researchers gave acidophilus (the good bacteria) to women during pregnancy, and to their babies after birth. The babies had a 50 percent lower chance of developing asthma compared with a control group.

We consider inflammation such an important part of our work because it's one of the first dominoes to fall on the path to serious conditions. Inflammation is a silent killer. Most people who have it don't know it. But it's important to uncover it, and treat it before a disease occurs, so you can prevent the disease from ever happening.

⋆　　⋆　　⋆

Some of the newest and most powerful drugs (which also have potentially serious side effects) are those that have been designed to target and suppress inflammatory cytokines.

Cytokines, proteins that dash around your body causing mischief, are the chemical messengers of your immune system, much as hormones are the messengers of your endocrine system, or neurotransmitters are the messengers of your nervous system.

Our immune system manufactures and releases these cytokines to alert the cells of our immune system to the presence of a threat. This could be an infection, or some other source of inflammation. Cytokines spread the message *inflammation!* like a smoke signal throughout our bodies, alerting other organs and cells of the immune system. Any therapy that blocks this signal reduces the extent of inflammation.

When cytokines get their signals straight, the forces that reduce and increase inflammation are in check. We want that fire when we have an infection, or an injury, to speed the healing process. But when the cytokines that create inflammation become overly dominant, all the diseases noted above can occur, as well as a process that leads to rapid aging of every part of the body.

What does this mean? We need to balance the cytokines—they are forces of inflammation. We can't avoid them, but by following ultraprevention, we will keep them in balance and prevent heart disease, stroke, dementia, diabetes, asthma, and all the other conditions that ultraprevention can forestall.

# FORCE 4: IMPAIRED DETOXIFICATION, OR WASTE

These days, when most of us hear the word *detoxification,* we think of celebrities checking into expensive resorts to deal with alcohol and drug abuse.

The truth is that all of us have detoxification problems. That's because detoxification is the process of breaking down and eliminating from the body anything that shouldn't be in it. It's a set of normal bodily functions that help your body stay healthy when it is exposed to harmful substances, either external or internal. Your body converts these toxic substances into nontoxic ones and excretes them.

If detoxification isn't functioning properly, excess waste accumulates in your body. It's similar to what happens when garbage collectors don't pick up the garbage off the streets. The waste piles high, making the neighborhood smell bad and creating the potential for illness.

Why does our body have to detoxify at all? Ages ago our diet was all natural. There were no pesticides, additives, or artificial colorings that needed to be removed. Nevertheless, the detoxification process developed in mammals long before humans evolved because of the need to eliminate the natural, normal compounds produced in the mammalian body. These compounds are by-products of chemicals the body secretes to perform a specific action for a limited duration of time. Detoxification also eliminates foreign, potentially toxic compounds often unavoidably ingested with our food.

Hormones are some of the natural substances that must be detoxified. After all, we don't use our old hormones over and over. The body constantly generates new ones, so the old ones must be eliminated to make room for them.

For example, your pituitary gland makes a hormone called ACTH that sends messages to the adrenal glands. Once the ACTH has done its job, it must leave your body—and that requires detoxification. Or the ovaries produce the hormone estrogen, which helps thicken the uterine lining and prepare a woman's breasts for a cycle of fertility. When that cycle ends, the estrogen has completed its purpose and must be eliminated.

Also needing detoxification are the waste products of metabolism, including the by-products of internal combustion discussed earlier, and cellular waste products such as carbon dioxide and water. Medications, too, must be detoxified. After a drug has done its work, it must leave your body, as must anything you ingest that your body doesn't need, such as food preservatives, or colorings, or pesticides. There are many plants containing poisonous and potentially lethal compounds that our body must detoxify if we accidentally ingest them (from poisonous mushrooms to poisonous roots, seeds, and leaves). Many unnatural substances, such as benzene, aflatoxin, PCBs, dioxin, and many pesticides, are carcinogenic (cancer-causing). We must eliminate them, too, as quickly as possible.

In order to detoxify the body, the body first has to make these substances water-soluble. That's because the wastes that we excrete—urine, sweat, and feces—are also water-based and the toxins exit through these routes.

Not everything in the body can be made water-soluble. Just as oil and water don't mix, neither do fat and blood. Blood is a water-based fluid. Fat, cholesterol, triglycerides, and hormones are lipid-based, which means that they dissolve when mixed with fat solvents such as ether or chloroform. Because fat is a form of energy storage, we don't tend to eliminate it from the body. It stays around for a long time (as most people who look at their abdomens have probably noticed).

Whatever the substance to be removed, the physical process of detoxification involves the chemical alteration of that substance to make it water-soluble for excretion in urine, sweat, or feces, or to package it for elimination in the bile.

(Detoxification and excretion are slightly different. Excretion refers to eliminating all unnecessary compounds from the body via stool, urine, sweat, breath, skin shedding, and hair growth. Detoxification refers to what happens *before* they can be excreted.)

Detoxification actually takes place in every cell of the body. And every cell is capable of transforming some compounds so that the body may more readily excrete them.

But few of us do a great job detoxifying ourselves. Sometimes it's a matter of genetics—some people are born excellent waste eliminators, while others aren't. A story that made headlines recently concerned a ten-year-old boy who, after a psychiatric evaluation, was put on a standard dose of Prozac. When this didn't seem to work, the doctor upped his dosage. But then the child began to react strangely, although the doctor determined it wasn't due to the medication. Then the child died. His parents were jailed, because the boy's autopsy showed he had astronomically high levels of Prozac in his bloodstream, and authorities assumed his parents had overdosed him. But a smart pathologist figured out that the poor boy didn't have the ability to process the drug; he died from a quantity of Prozac that might not have even registered on someone else.

Our ability to detoxify is also influenced by the level of toxins we're exposed to. The body has a limited capacity to do all this detoxification. If you've been exposed to a large quantity of toxins, the body can become overwhelmed and may run out of the nutrients it needs to perform properly.

Another variable in our ability to detoxify are enzymes, on which our detoxification system relies for its work. They are the catalysts that make possible all of the body's chemical reactions.

There are thousands of enzymes living inside of our cells, particularly in the liver. The liver is the workhorse of our detoxification system. In fact, it contains a myriad of different enzymes expressly designed to catalyze, or generate, the specific chemical reactions that allow our bodies to eliminate waste products.

As mentioned, every cell in your body has some capacity to detoxify. But the reason the liver handles the lion's share of the job is due to its location. The liver sits right between the digestive tract and the bloodstream. Nothing can get into the bloodstream from the digestive tract without first passing through the liver. So anything we swallow has to be processed by the liver before it moves on.

The liver is constantly asking itself: "Is this something I should let into the bloodstream?" and "Is this something that I should detoxify?" If you swallow something that shouldn't get into your bloodstream, such as an artificial preservative, the liver will recognize it and say, "This is not food. I don't want this to get into the bloodstream. Instead I'll trap it and keep it here so I can detoxify and eliminate it."

Every organ has some capability to detoxify, however. For example, the lungs breathe in good air and exhale bad air, ridding the body of waste products that are gaseous, including carbon dioxide and methane.

The kidneys, too, detoxify, by constantly filtering our blood. They filter out the bad stuff we want eliminated in the urine from needed substances like nutrients, which we want to retain.

The skin also plays a role in detoxification, because it excretes sweat, which also eliminates compounds we don't need or want in the body. Similarly, the skin tries not to excrete things that we do want, like proteins. If you sweated protein, you would develop malnutrition.

★   ★   ★

If the body is not detoxifying properly, undesirable substances may accumulate, causing symptoms that can lead to serious illness.

Some of the more common problems related to poor detoxification are fatigue (as well as the more serious chronic fatigue syndrome), pain, chronic hormonal problems (including PMS), fibroids, and heavy menstrual bleeding. Both Parkinson's and Alzheimer's diseases are also linked to detoxification abnormalities.

Parkinson's is a classic example of a disease caused by a combination of a genetic predisposition and exposure to a toxin—usually a petrochemical-derived toxin such as a chemical solvent, ink, or pesticide. This is why farmers, with their high exposure to pest-killing chemicals, are documented as having some of the highest rates of this disease of any occupation.

Victims of Parkinson's suffer a buildup of these partially detoxified compounds, which in turn light a fire of inflammation in the brain, creating oxidative stress, or free radicals; these destroy a part of the brain that controls movement. This is why tremors are one of the major symptoms of Parkinson's.

About two decades ago an epidemic of Parkinson's occurred among teenagers in Southern California. Such an outbreak was previously unheard of, but investigators quickly detected a common link: All of the teens had taken the same chemistry class, in which their professor had showed them how to synthesize the drug Demerol. Apparently the kids went right home to make it themselves in their bathrooms.

But they didn't get the chemical reaction exactly right. Instead of making Demerol, they made a compound called MPTP, which is similar to Demerol except that, unlike Demerol, the body can't eliminate it. The teens all woke up the next morning with Parkinson's disease—and it wasn't a temporary Parkinson's that would pass as soon as the drug wore off; it was the progressive, lethal condition. Just a few years ago the first two victims died from the disease; when authorities completed their autopsies, they indeed found an ongoing inflammation in the brain caused by the MPTP taken eighteen years earlier.

The *Journal of the American Medical Association* (vol. 279, page 1200) reported that in 1998 there were 104,000 deaths due to drug reactions, as well as 2.5 million serious adverse reactions requiring prolonged hospitalization. Such tragedies were not the result of mistakes, or overdoses, or drugs given for the wrong reason—these drugs were prescribed and dispensed properly by trained doctors and nurses. No, almost all of these incidents were related to detoxification problems.

Despite all this, conventional Western medicine has been slow to recognize detoxification as a significant area of study. In part, this is because reliable laboratory tools to assess detoxification levels have only recently become available. But because the study of detoxification is new, it isn't taught in medical school. The average doctor knows little about it.

The one aspect of detoxification widely studied today is in regard to toxins found in the environment. One of the most interesting examples: Science has known for several years that affluent women are much more prone to breast cancer than women of lower social and economic classes. This surprised researchers, because there was no way to explain how breast cancer could know what your bank account looks like.

The initial explanation was that women with more money often have fewer children; they are more apt to have careers, to have had a greater number of menstrual cycles for a longer period of time, and are less apt to have nursed. (The connection: Levels of certain sex hormones are known to promote, or protect against, reproductive cancers.)

But although this may be true, such reasons only account for about 10 percent of those additional cases of cancer among affluent women. How do we account for the other 90 percent?

The answer may lie in their lifestyle. Another difference between more and less affluent women is that when the former's clothes get dirty, they are more likely to send them to the dry cleaner than do the scrubbing themselves. At the cleaner, the clothes become laden with toxic chemicals that are absorbed into the body and have to be detoxified.

Furthermore, when wealthy women's lawns start sprouting weeds, they do not go outside to weed and fertilize; they call in a lawn maintenance company to do the job with a combination pesticide–fertilizer–weed killer that contains a mixture of toxic chemicals. So it may be the environment in which these women place themselves that leads to cancer, as much as their reproductive history.

Because toxicity often affects the liver, we must consider it a detoxification problem whenever blood tests show that the liver is abnormal. Likewise, toxicity often interferes with the brain. Think about the various chemicals we put into our bodies (from caffeine and alcohol to sedatives and antihistamines) and their impact on our minds and moods—until our bodies eliminate or detoxify the offending agents.

The reason the effects of alcohol or caffeine eventually wear off is that the liver has finally cleared the substance out of the blood-stream. The same is true for the effects of medications, or the harmful effects of poisons, carcinogens, or other toxins.

Impaired detoxification causes many recognizable conditions besides Parkinson's and breast cancer. These include damage from the statin drugs (such as Mevacor, Lipitor, Zocor, and Pravachol, prescribed to lower cholesterol), Reye's syndrome (a potentially lethal disorder that occurs when someone with impaired detoxification of aspirin takes it for a virus), or the fatal liver failure caused by the diabetes drug Rezulin, which was associated with the death of at least sixty-three people before it was withdrawn in March 2000.

At Canyon Ranch, where we consider detoxification a critical area of testing and treatment, we ask our patients about certain symptoms they may have—everything from fatigue to skin rash from medication allergies to sensitivity to particular foods or substances.

We also perform a special test in which we give patients small amounts of three substances: aspirin, caffeine, and acetaminophen. The next day we look in their blood, urine, and saliva to see if the drugs were all processed well and completely eliminated.

Improper handling of one of these compounds by the body reveals an imbalance in detoxification that can often be remedied by providing the liver with the appropriate nutrients or supplements to enhance its detoxification function.

The body needs many nutrients for proper detoxification. So if we discover problems in this area, we recommend several remedies: the sulfur-containing amino acids, found in foods such as broccoli, brussels sprouts, cabbage, cauliflower, kale, bok choy, garlic, and onion; vitamins, such as vitamin A, vitamins $B_6$ and $B_{12}$, and folic acid; and/or trace minerals such as magnesium, selenium, zinc, copper, and manganese. Many plant compounds, or phytonutrients, are also powerful detoxifiers, such as those found in silymarin, derived from a milk thistle plant.

By supporting the liver and reducing its burden of detoxification, we can promote its long-term healthy function, because it is one of the organs vital for longevity. And by addressing and promoting detoxification in general, we can eliminate one of the basic underlying mechanisms of many illnesses and diseases, and prevent those disorders from developing.

# FORCE 5: OXIDATIVE STRESS, OR RUST

When metal rusts, it's a sign of the chemical process known as oxidation. Rusting indicates the damage incurred by exposure to oxygen; we say the metal is becoming oxidized. Here oxygen steals electrons away from the metal; this changes the properties of that metal, as well as its appearance.

Another example of oxidation takes place when you bite into an apple and leave it on a table; the fruit will soon turn brown as it's exposed to more oxygen.

Because the properties of nature operate similarly inside and outside our bodies, this process also occurs when oxygen comes into contact with the body's tissues—oxygen steals electrons away from those tissues, changing and, unfortunately, damaging them. They become oxidized, just as metal does when it rusts.

Every one of us has, and needs, millions of oxidants in our body. However, oxidant molecules can cause injury to our tissues whenever they are present in excess, becoming a source of illness, causing oxidative stress. This phenomenon was first noted in 1954 by Dr. Denham Harmon, an organic chemist at the University of California, Berkeley. Dr. Harmon theorized that oxidants were the cause of aging, as well as the major cause of most diseases. His theory has continued to hold up and has received substantial verification over the past half century.

Our bodies thrive on oxygen: We breathe it, and then use it in the process of combustion to burn fuel to make energy (as we saw in the section on metabolism). But this use of oxygen for our cellular metabolism has a by-product: waste in the form of high-energy oxygen molecules that are highly flammable and tend to "burn" any tissue they come into contact with.

These reactive oxygen molecules are also known as free radicals. (They're called this because one of many definitions for the word *radical* refers to a "root" cause, and free radicals are formed by the splitting of a parent, or root, compound.) These free radicals cause damage to cellular structures and tissues, and this damage is what we call oxidative stress—the stress put on our bodies by the use of oxygen.

Most of the conditions that we associate with aging, such as wrinkles, heart disease, and Alzheimer's, are related to excess oxidative stress in the body. As Dr. Harmon stated, "Very few individuals, if any, reach their potential maximum life span; they die instead prematurely of a wide variety of diseases—the vast majority being 'free radical' diseases."

Although Dr. Harmon's research is a half-century old, the public has become familiar with his concept only recently. This is partly because conventional medicine, now that it has recognized the phenomenon, has become fascinated with it—in the last five years more than five thousand articles on the subject have appeared in research journals.

And until recently, tests to measure levels of oxidative stress were available only to research centers. The good news is that this situation has changed—today commercial labs will conduct the test through an over-the-counter urine test available at drugstores, meaning anyone can check his or her oxidative stress level. Still, most people haven't yet done this.

They should, because some of us have unhealthy levels but don't know it—and know it we must. This is because free radicals are generated whenever and wherever energy is produced—which is mainly inside our mitochondria.

If you recall from the discussion on page 193, the mitochondria resemble tiny balloons filled with energy-producing enzymes. As these little balloons make energy, free radicals are created and released. If the mitochondria don't sponge up these free radicals quickly, they can travel to the surface of the balloon and cause damage to the membranes surrounding the mitochondria, even punching holes in them, whereupon the contents of the mitochondria start to leak out.

The mitochondria then lose the important chemicals and enzymes that allow them to produce energy. This process is the beginning of the end for a mitochondrion, and its useful function soon ceases.

Once this loss had occurred, the body must then attempt to repair the damage. That, too, requires energy, which means there's less energy available for all the normal things your body should be doing. Oxidative stress throws a monkey wrench in your body's metabolism, because now your metabolism can't do what it is supposed to, which is create energy.

Moreover, part of that repair process may lead to activation of the immune system—and damage not just to the cells, but to the organs themselves, because the inflammation that occurs in response to free radicals is harmful. Inflammation is one of the ways tissues in the body are injured.

Almost every organ can be susceptible to damage from oxidative stress. And the symptoms are countless, including fatigue, muscle weakness, muscle and joint pain, digestive problems, anxiety, depression, itchy skin, headaches, as well as trouble concentrating and trouble fighting infections.

The most common diseases triggered by oxidative stress include heart disease, cancer, osteoarthritis, rheumatoid arthritis, diabetes, and neurodegenerative problems like Alzheimer's, Parkinson's, and multiple sclerosis. It can also lead to chronic fatigue, chemical sensitivity, and fibromyalgia.

Research has shown that almost all illnesses have an increased level of oxidative stress as a common thread.

In fact, oxidative stress is the common end of most disease processes. A recent article in the *Journal of the American Medical Association* (October 23, 2002) ties together problems with impaired metabolism (insulin resistance and abdominal obesity), inflammation, and oxidative stress. Researchers found that women who had more fat around the middle due to insulin resistance also had more inflammation and oxidative stress, causing thicker blood and more clotting (the main reason people get heart attacks or strokes). When these women lost the weight around the middle, their insulin level went down, and they had less inflammation and less oxidative stress.

One of the chief causes of oxidative stress is, surprisingly and unfortunately, the processing by your body of the food you eat. As we've noted, when you process food, you digest it and turn it into fuel, which is then burned inside the mitochondria (in the process of internal combustion) to make energy. You're also generating free radicals when you do this. This is normal, and is why our bodies naturally manufacture antioxidants every day, just to douse those free radical sparks.

The problem occurs when the quantity of free radicals we generate from processing food exceeds the body's ability to quench them. This is most likely to occur when your food intake is excessive, particularly of foods with a lot of empty calories. Eating meals or snacks high in calories, but low in antioxidants, contributes to increasing the level of oxidative stress in our bodies.

Studies in which rats are restricted in their calorie intake (but not in their nutrient intake) have repeatedly shown that these animals live up to 40 percent longer than rats allowed to eat as usual. And not only do these calorie-restricted rats live longer, they also live better; that is, they are protected from developing the usual diseases of aging, such as arthritis, diabetes, dementia, and cancer. They also look great (well, as great as a rat can look), with thick, shiny coats, full sets of whiskers, and shiny eyes. On top of that, they can run through the mazes as well as younger rats.

Some of the best human evidence of the calorie-reduction concept sprang from the Biosphere II experiments. Here eight men and women lived in a self-sustaining enclosed environment in the Arizona desert for two years, growing or raising all their own food, producing their own oxygen, making their own water, and processing their own waste. Because the amount of food they could produce was limited, they ended up on a calorie-restricted diet.

After the two years were up, the men had lost about 18 percent of their body weight; the women had lost 10 percent. And, every measurable variable (body fat, blood pressure, exercise capacity, oxygen consumption, blood sugar levels, cholesterols, cortisol levels, white blood counts, and so on) showed by every measurable parameter that these people had become substantially younger than when they entered the environment two years earlier.

The reason for this? By consuming fewer calories, they experienced a much lower level of oxidative stress.

Sources of oxidative stress can be both internal and external. The external ones include exposure to any kind of environmental pollution, petrochemicals, or heavy metals.

There are also lifestyle-related causes of oxidative stress, such as smoking, drinking alcohol, excessive exercise, prescription drugs, and especially overeating. Trying too hard to get a tan can also hurt; too much sun (ultraviolet radiation) contributes to oxidative stress.

Internal sources of oxidative stress include infections, whether acute or chronic, as well as problems with blood sugar regulation. We've talked about insulin resistance before and here it is again: Problems with sugar imbalance lead to increased free radicals.

Nutritional deficiencies also contribute to oxidative stress—if we're selenium deficient, or if we don't have enough vitamin E or vitamin A or other key antioxidants, we may not be able to supply our body with the needed factors that will keep our antioxidant system working. Being overweight, too, can hurt. Fat tissues produce inflammatory molecules that lead to increased oxidative stress.

We find that oxidative stress and inflammation are closely linked. It seems that wherever you find one, you'll find the other. Take an area where there's a lot of oxidative stress—for example, a smoker's lungs. The smoke is an oxidant, because it's burned tobacco, and thus highly oxidized. When the lungs absorb that oxidized tobacco, damage occurs to the lung tissue, which soon causes inflammation. This is why smokers get bronchitis—the suffix *-itis* means inflammation, and bronchitis is inflammation of the bronchial tubes.

Oxidative stress doesn't always need to be tested—especially if you're already ill, because if you are, you're definitely suffering from oxidative stress. It is a basic mechanism in all sickness.

At Canyon Ranch we test for oxidative stress in patients whom we might not otherwise suspect are ill. But if we discover someone does have a high level of oxidative stress, it's a sign that intervention is necessary to prevent future disease. At this point we recommend changes in diet, lifestyle, and nutrients and supplements.

One of the main reasons the government (and your mother) tells you to eat more fruits and vegetables is because they contain a whole range of antioxidants, such as vitamins C and E, and beta-carotene, as well as flavonoids and other powerful chemicals.

We also recommend vitamins to support the liver, such as the B vitamins; minerals including magnesium, choline, and lecithin; and certain foods, including garlic, onions, broccoli, cabbage, brussels sprouts, kale, and cauliflower.

This brings up what we call the NCR concept. We believe we should all be eating foods with a high nutrient-to-calorie ratio, or NCR. We want our patients to eat foods that offer many nutrients, but not many calories. When a diet is predominantly composed of foods that are high in calories but low in nutrients, you will find a high level of oxidative stress. These foods include that much-discussed white menace: white sugar, white flour and white bread, white pasta, and white rice, as well as pure carbohydrates, starches, and sweeteners.

On the other hand, foods that are unrefined are quite high in the important nutrients. Your best choice: fruits and vegetables. (It's not hard to tell which fruits and vegetables have the highest nutrient quantity; they're usually the most colorful. The color occurs because they are full of antioxidants like carotene, lycopene, lutein, xanthine, proanthocyandins, and xeanthins.)

In order to process the food we eat, we need all of the specific nutrients that are normally found in high-NCR foods; these prevent oxidative stress. That's why it's better to eat whole wheat or whole grain bread instead of white bread made from refined flour. You will gain the benefit of the B vitamins, vitamin E, and the other vitamins and minerals found within the whole foods.

# TESTING THE FIVE FORCES OF ILLNESS

Recent years have seen an explosive growth in commercial laboratories offering specialized testing in various aspects of the five forces. This testing can be helpful in identifying which of these forces are present, and to what degree. There are many tests that you can take; below is just a sample of what is available.

Many of these tests can be ordered from the same commercial labs used by your doctor's office or local hospital. The others are run primarily by specialty labs.

These tests are often of the blood, but a few test urine, and these can be done at home and mailed to the lab in special mailers provided by the labs.

Most tests will have to be ordered by a doctor. Each lab provides some interpretation of the results, although your results should always be reviewed with a physician to interpret them in the context of your overall health. To learn more about how to obtain these tests, how to interpret them, and what to do about abnormal results, please go to our website, www.ultraprevention.com.

Some of the tests that we find helpful include the following. Please note that:

A (1) denotes tests usually run by big commercial labs, including Quest (800-842-7412; www.questdiagnostics.com), Labcorp (800-886-4073; www.labcorp.com), Unilab (818-996-7300; www.unilab.com), and Dynacare (972-387-3200; www.dynacare.com).

A (2) denotes tests usually run by specialty labs such as Doctor's

Data (800-323-2784; www.doctorsdata.com), Great Smokies Diagnostic Lab (800-522-4762; www.gsdl.com), ImmunoLab (800-231-9197; www.immunolabs.com), ImmunoSciences Lab (800-950-4686; www.immno-sci-lab.com), Metametrix Lab (800-221-4640; www.metametrix.com), and others.

### TESTING FOR SLUDGE

Homocysteine: You can test the level of this amino acid in the bloodstream. Ideal levels are less than 9. (1)

Essential fatty acid levels: The levels of essential fatty acids can be measured in the blood, specifically in the red blood cells themselves. This measures the levels of omega-3, omega-6, and other fatty acids directly. (1)

Red blood cell minerals: Levels of minerals such as magnesium, selenium, iodine, zinc, and copper can be measured in the red blood cells. (1)

Methylmalonic acid (blood or urine): High levels are a sensitive indicator of vitamin $B_{12}$ deficiency. (1)

A stool analysis can determine digestion and absorption; this can identify if foods are either not being broken down and digested properly, or not being absorbed—i.e., if meat fibers or fats are seen in your stool, you are not properly breaking down meat or absorbing fat. (2)

### TESTING FOR BURNOUT
### Testing for Mitochondrial Malfunction

Urinary organic acids: Measurement of acidic compounds in the urine provides a rich amount of information about nutritional aspects of cellular energy production. (2)

Cardiometabolic stress testing: Measuring oxygen consumption during exercise (VO2 max) is an excellent way of assessing our mitochondria's metabolic capacity.

## Testing for Insulin Resistance

An insulin response test measures the insulin response to a fixed dosage of sugar (75 grams of glucose taken orally). Before and two hours after drinking the glucose drink, the blood levels of insulin and glucose determine how sensitive (or resistant) the body is to the effects of insulin. We feel that normal insulin values at two hours are less than 25, and a normal glucose level is less than 140. (1)

Lipid profile (total cholesterol, LDL, HDL, triglycerides): A triglyceride level over 150 or a triglyceride-to-HDL ratio greater than 4.3 are highly suggestive of insulin resistance, as is an HDL level of less than 40 in men or less than 50 in women. (1)

Waist-hip ratio: This low-tech test is surprisingly accurate. Simply divide your waist measurement (at the belly button level) by the hip measurement (at the widest point over your hips). For women, your number should be 0.8 or less; for men, less than 0.9. Higher values are associated with insulin resistance. (Also be wary if your waist is over 36 inches in women or 45 inches in men.)

## Testing for Thyroid Dysfunction

TSH, or thyroid stimulating hormone, is produced by the pituitary gland and can be measured in the blood. Normal levels are between 0.3 and 3.5, although 1.0 to 2.0 may be optimal. (1)

Free T4 and free T3: Direct measurement of thyroid hormone levels in the blood in conjunction with the TSH level provide helpful information regarding thyroid function. (1)

Thyroid antibodies: Thyroid peroxidase antibodies and anti-thyroglobulin antibodies can detect people at risk of developing hypothyroidism (underactive thyroid) because of the presence of antibodies directed against the thyroid gland. (1)

Resting metabolic rate: Measurement of our basal, or resting, metabolic rate using sophisticated equipment can sometimes be a clue to the presence of an underactive thyroid gland. (1)

## TESTING FOR HEAT

C-reactive protein: The best test here is called the high-sensitivity CRP, also known as the "Cardio CRP," which is a more accurate test than the standard CRP. Optimal levels should be 0.7 or less. Acceptable levels range up to 2. (1)

Sedimentation (sed) rate: This is a little less accurate than the CRP test, but high sed rates are signs of inflammation. Normal values are less than 20. (1)

Fibrinogen level: Fibrinogen, one of the chief constituents involved in clotting, is made by the liver. Fibrinogen rises in response to inflammation, and is measured in the blood. (1)

Food allergy tests: By measuring levels of antibodies (IgG, IgE) in the blood to a battery of different foods, potentially reactive foods can be identified with a single blood test. (2)

Gluten/celiac disease: Specific tests to check for gluten (primarily in wheat) allergy include the anti-gliadin antibody test, and the tissue transglutaminase assay, both measured in the blood. (1)

Tests for infections: A number of tests can be used to detect hidden infections, including antibody tests (e.g., antibodies to Lyme disease, *Helicobacter pylori,* or HIV). These look for antibodies to specific germs. Tests are also available that look directly for the germ itself, rather than the antibody. These include PCR tests and cultures. (1,2)

## TESTING FOR WASTE

Detoxification challenge test: By measuring the body's ability to clear a fixed dosage of specific substances, we can learn about a person's ability to detoxify and eliminate some chemicals. During this test, we measure how someone's liver is able to clear fixed quantities of caffeine, aspirin, and acetaminophen. A small dose of each is given on one day, and the next day we measure what by-products are found in the blood and urine. Delayed or impaired detoxification in specific areas can point to nutritional deficiencies involved in detoxification, or weak enzyme systems in the liver that could be assisted with specific foods or supplements. (2)

Blood reduced glutathione: One of the most powerful detoxifiers, the level of reduced glutathione measured in the blood provides information about this critical compound. (2)

Hair analysis: As a screening test for heavy metal toxicity, hair analysis can give clues to the body's burden of metals such as mercury, arsenic, lead, and cadmium. Hair analysis is not accurate for assessment of general nutrition, however. (2)

Urinary organic acids: Measurement of certain acidic compounds in the urine can provide information about the body's ability to detoxify certain solvents as well as some hormones and carcinogens. (2)

## TESTING FOR RUST

Lipid peroxides are oxidized fats. Measuring the level of these oxidized fats in the blood or urine provides an index of the body's antioxidant status. (2)

Superoxide dismutase (SOD), glutathione peroxidase (GSHPx), and catalase: These are three of the most important natural antioxidant enzymes. The levels of these antioxidants can be directly measured in the blood. (2)

Glutathione: The levels of this important antioxidant can also be directly measured in the blood. (2)

Urinary hydroxyl markers: Levels of free radicals such as catechol and 2,3-dihydroxybenzoate are measured after an aspirin and acetaminophen challenge, and provide information about how well our bodies absorb or quench free radicals after detoxification of aspirin or acetaminophen. (2)

Blood antioxidant levels: Levels of vitamin A, vitamin E, coenzyme Q10, and beta-carotene can be directly measured in the blood. (1,2)

★   ★   ★

Addressing sludge, burnout, heat, waste, and rust are the backbone of our ultraprevention system. Yet most doctors don't pay attention to any of these forces because they operate under this model: If it ain't broke, don't fix it. The problem is that "it" may well be broken already. But most doctors don't realize this, because they wait until something is damaged almost beyond repair before they act.

Knowledge of these five forces gives us an advantage over other doctors. They allow us a lead time. By looking for telltale signs regarding these processes before diseases develop, we can prevent them from occurring.

This means that if you, too, are willing to pay attention to the five forces of illness, you are much more likely to remain healthy than if you don't. It's difficult for us to believe that everyone isn't already doing this. It isn't that hard, and it can possibly make your life a great deal better—or even save it.

Still, we hear our patients rationalize, "Even if we did know about these five forces, isn't it up to our doctors, not us, to do something about them?"

The answer to that is a resounding "No!"

It's up to you. One of the greatest changes taking place in our medical system is the empowerment of the patient. We believe everyone should become his or her own health advocate. If you sit around waiting for your doctor to catch up with ultraprevention, you'll endanger your health.

Why would you want to do that? Why not grasp the power to do everything you can to remain healthy?

Anyone and everyone reading this book should ask their doctor to test for these five forces. Get checked for inflammation, obtain a detoxification profile, and so on. If your doctor is unfamiliar with these tests, please go to www.ultraprevention.com to learn more about how and when to take them.

And every one of you should follow as much of the plan in Part III as you feel makes sense. By doing so, you will have a chance to become more fit and more healthy than you may have ever thought possible.

You will also uncover your own innate good health, which will become the foundation on which you can build a full and vigorous life. And you will be able to take advantage of the most powerful scientific discoveries of our time, made practical and easy to understand. Our program will allow you to protect, energize, and renew both body and mind, giving you the best chance to reach your optimum health.

To hell with trying to live longer. Our goal isn't life span. It's health span. Life span just means staying alive. We want people to stay alive healthily. Our goal is to take the life span, divide by the health span, and make that number as close to one as possible.

Today we stand at the beginning of an entirely new era of medicine, one in which people create their own good health through a carefully developed system that helps them and their doctors identify those areas where they are at risk, and correct them before that risk develops into actual distress. The key to ultraprevention: You don't have to wait until you are sick to get well.

As a result, we believe that what we now call ultraprevention will become, in a few decades, the standard practice of medicine. This is why ultraprevention is the future—tomorrow's medicine, today.

# PART III

# The Six-Week Ultraprevention Plan

To fight a disease after it has occurred is like trying to dig a well when one is thirsty or forging a weapon once a war has begun.
—*The Yellow Emperor's Classic of Internal Medicine*

# THE SIX-WEEK PLAN: REMOVE, REPAIR, RECHARGE

During the next six weeks, you can unlearn a lifetime of habits that have been slowly creating the five forces of illness:

- Malnutrition, or sludge
- Impaired metabolism, or burnout
- Inflammation, or heat
- Impaired detoxification, or waste
- Oxidative stress, or rust

You will also learn a new set of habits that will correct and eliminate each one of these forces, bringing your health back into balance as you restore energy and vitality. At the end of the six weeks you may not find yourself in sudden and miraculous perfect health, but you will find that you have learned how to take care of yourself in the best possible way for the rest of your life. And some of you will, indeed, feel dramatically better!

As you read, please bear the following in mind: In this plan we will suggest certain practices, foods, or programs more than once. When dealing with such a holistic topic as health, it's simply impossible not to re-cover the same ground when talking about different subject matter—for instance, we will ask you in several places to consider an elimination diet. That's because such a diet can do many things: It can help you identify allergies, it can optimize your digestive system, it can reduce oxidative stress, and so on.

Likewise, we mention the need for exercise in several different contexts. Again, exercise is important for more than one reason. Rather than exclude it from the plan after the first time it's been mentioned, we've decided to let you know each time exercise can help—in each different manner. This way, you will have even more motivation to go out and do it.

We also refer to several parts of the plan more than once, because we don't expect you to do everything in the exact order we recommend. We do not believe that one general prescription can fit all. Likewise, we don't believe a book can tell all its readers exactly what to eat, how to exercise, or what to think, because each of you is different. Each of you has a different metabolism, a different body type, a different genetic composition, and different desires for your life. With that in mind, our program is designed to steer you in the right direction—and help you stay there.

Another important point to bear in mind: Few of you will be able to follow every one of our recommendations. Frankly, even we can't, and don't, follow every single piece of advice listed. Instead, we hope you will simply do your best. Try what you can. Do what seems right. And if something feels wrong to you, if your body tells you to stop, trust your instincts.

You may also note that at times we seem to offer contradictory advice. For example, we say that eggs are a great source of many nutrients and vitamins, including selenium and vitamin $B_6$; their sulfur content also helps the liver detoxify. We also suggest you try an elimination diet to avoid them. The point is that some of you may have discovered that eggs trigger allergies or inflammation, so you should search out other sources of the nutrients they contain. On the other hand, if your system thrives on eggs, include them in your diet. Be sensible. Again, not every recommendation will work for every reader. Just because eggs are potentially damaging to some doesn't mean the rest of you should avoid them.

We are proposing the following as a six-week plan. You'll start thinking about, and working on, the material in Step One for the first two weeks. For the next two weeks, you'll add the material in Step Two. Then you'll begin including the material in Step Three.

Although we wouldn't encourage you to move through the program more quickly, if you decide you want more time to incorporate as many of these recommendations as possible into your life, take it. This is not a drill. This is not a test. This is life. The ultraprevention plan is a guide to help you improve your health. The more you enjoy the plan, and the more comfortable you feel with it, the more likely you are to heed it.

Of course, the ultimate enjoyment comes with the increased sense of energy and health you will feel as the elements of the plan become an integral part of your life.

## STEP ONE: REMOVE

Central to this first phase of our six-week program is a concept called "total load."

Think of your body as an empty pitcher that is constantly being filled with the cumulative burden of harmful and potentially dangerous substances such as carcinogens, anti-nutrients, allergens, oxidants, and the waste products of your own metabolism.

There is a small spigot at the bottom of the pitcher draining these harmful things (representing the many natural processes your body uses to heal and soothe itself, from detoxification to the immune response). But if the flow is too slow, or if the pitcher fills up faster than it empties, at some point the pitcher will begin to overflow. At that point, symptoms occur and disease appears.

No one specific item listed below will necessarily tip the balance. It's the cumulative effect of all exposures and influences, the total load that places excessive stress on our bodies' capacity for health. Ultimately, our natural healing ability becomes overwhelmed and illness appears. Genetics and organ reserve play key roles in determining your susceptibility to disease—that is, how much the pitcher can hold before it overflows. But so does how you manage what enters and leaves that pitcher.

The two-week remove phase of our ultraprevention plan is designed to stop the rate at which that pitcher is being filled.

## STEP TWO: REPAIR

Once we have removed the impediments to health, we can begin to heal and repair the damage from our past. The repair process provides us with the raw materials our bodies use to heal and energize. Promoting optimal nutrition and an efficient metabolism accelerates the repair process. So does fighting inflammation, enhancing detoxification, and stopping rust.

In Step Two, you'll learn how to revise your eating habits to deal with nutritional deficiencies. You will also learn how to repair the intestinal tract, the key interface between the world and your immune system. We'll detail ways to support and nourish the immune system, enhance detoxification (our inner garbage-disposal system), and protect the body from oxidative stress, the internal rusting process that leads to accelerated aging. And we'll explain how to mobilize the hormonal troops that supervise almost every vital function of the body.

This phase will infuse energy and life back into your cells, as vital as a baby's first breath. During this two-week phase you will remember how good it feels to feel good.

## STEP THREE: RECHARGE

Overcoming the five forces of illness also involves working on deeper levels of healing that we refer to collectively as recharge.

This process involves more subtle activities, but ones that nonetheless have a huge impact on your physiological and biochemical functioning.

Recharging activities include creating a regular rhythm of restful sleep, moving your body, correcting physical problems, creatively managing stress, and building a life with meaning and purpose. During this two-week phase, you will learn lifelong techniques to help you recharge your body and enhance your overall health.

# STEP ONE: REMOVE—
# THE FIRST TWO WEEKS

**GOALS:**
1. CLEAR THE SLUDGE
2. ELIMINATE THE WASTE
3. REMOVE THE RUST
4. COOL THE HEAT
5. END THE BURNOUT

## 1. CLEAR THE SLUDGE

Remove anti-nutrients to overcome malnutrition and give your body the support it needs.

Anti-nutrients are compounds in food that can cause more harm than good when we eat them. Examples of anti-nutrients include hydrogenated and saturated fats, sugar, refined grains and starches, caffeine, alcohol, and carcinogens.

Here's how to remove anti-nutrients:

### Get an Oil Change

Go through your kitchen and throw out all foods whose ingredients list includes hydrogenated oil, or partially hydrogenated vegetable oil. The most common foods containing hydrogenated oils are margarine, crackers, chips, packaged baked goods, and store-bought snacks.

Eliminate all refined oils, including corn oil, safflower oil, sunflower oil, and soybean oil, which are primarily polyunsaturated

*good*

and are simply not as healthful as the monounsaturated oil found in olive oil. An exception may be unrefined canola oil, which does contain a high proportion of healthy monounsaturated oil.

When you shop for oil, look for expeller-pressed canola, which has not been extracted with solvents (such as hexane). This may mean buying your canola oil in a health food or specialty store rather than at your neighborhood supermarket, since the bulk of canola oil sold to grocery chains is solvent-extracted using chemicals, and then refined further in the process of bleaching and deodorizing. Small amounts of other unrefined oils are fine, including sesame, walnut, and other nut oils. *good*

Reduce your intake of saturated animal fat. This includes fat found in meats, butter, and dairy products. Saturated fats in general should be minimized, including vegetable sources of saturated fat such as coconut or palm oils.

Animal fat carries an additional risk—chemical toxins such as pesticides, PCBs, dioxins, and others are concentrated in animal fat, because these chemicals are fat-soluble. Whenever we eat beef or pork fat, we also consume whatever toxins the cow or pig ingested. When eating meat, choose lean cuts and always trim the fat.

## Eliminate the White Menace

By this we mean sugar—and anything our bodies can quickly convert to sugar. Learn to identify all forms of sugar. Try a sugar fast for these two weeks and see what happens. You're likely to feel more energetic and mentally sharp, less hungry, and you may even lose weight.

Here are some specifics on what to avoid:

### Sugar itself and sugary sweets

Read food labels to identify sugar in other disguises such as high-fructose corn syrup, sucrose, glucose, maltose, dextrose, lactose, fructose, corn syrup, or fruit juice concentrate. Food processors do not have to state if there is added sugar in their products. They must list only the total number of grams of sugar. But sugar is sugar by any other name, and that includes honey, barley malt, maple sugar, Sucanat, natural cane sugar, malt syrup, cornstarch, disaccharides, turbinado sugar, and molasses. Avoid hidden sugars in foods like ketchup, salad dressings, luncheon meats, canned fruits, bread, peanut butter, crackers, soups, sausage, yogurt, relish, cheese dips, chewing gum, breakfast cereals, and many more packaged and processed foods. In other words, the best way to keep your sugar intake low is to avoid taking in extra sugars in any form.

### White pasta, white bread, white rice, and white potatoes

Yes, pasta and white bread! Nothing seems to strike fear in our patients' hearts more than asking them to reduce or give up their bread and pasta. But as we've seen, our bodies can convert pasta and white bread into sugar in our bloodstream about as quickly as we can get table sugar into our bloodstream.

### Carbonated soft drinks, including diet drinks

These trick the body into craving more sweets. Even when they proclaim that they're part fruit juice, or that they're actually good for you, avoid them.

### Eliminate Excess Salt

Adding extra salt to food causes extra fluid retention. For every gram (1,000 mg) of sodium you eat, your body retains about ten ounces of water. Although our bodies require only about 500 mg of sodium per day, Americans eat on average seven or eight times that amount. Extra sodium raises the blood pressure and places extra strain on the heart and kidneys. It can also lead to osteoporosis (thinning of the bones), by causing loss of calcium in the urine.

We recommend sodium intake of less than 2,000 mg per day.
To reduce your salt intake:

• Minimize salt added to food, either at the table or when cooking.

• Avoid commercially produced or processed food.

• Avoid fast foods or junk food.

• Read labels carefully—choose low-sodium varieties whenever possible.

• Try using herbal substitutes or salt substitutes with potassium chloride (in moderation).

• Use herbs, spices, lemon, or lime rather than salt.

### Throw Out Processed Foods

Commercially prepared, packaged, and processed foods are often loaded with preservatives, artificial colorings, flavor enhancers, and sweeteners, not to mention hydrogenated fats and sodium. Do your best to follow our favorite motto: Buy fresh, eat fresh!

### Reduce Caffeine Intake

For an optimal response to our plan, we recommend eliminating or sharply reducing your caffeine intake. Caffeine raises levels of adrenaline, causes overexcitation, increases stress, and impairs the relaxation response. It's hard to be at peace when you're revved up on caffeine.

If you're a caffeine user, it's best to taper off slowly to avoid unpleasant withdrawal effects, particularly headaches.

Sources of caffeine include: coffee, black or green teas, colas and other soft drinks, chocolate and cocoa, and various medications for weight control, pain, menstrual pain relief, and colds. Because each medication is different, check the labels, where caffeine content will be listed.

### Remove Excess Animal Protein

Excess animal protein in your diet increases your levels of homocysteine, a harmful by-product of protein digestion. Excess animal protein also places added strain on the kidneys, which have to filter this excess protein. And it stresses your bones by leaching calcium from the skeleton.

Animal protein is accompanied by animal fat, an undesirable form of saturated fat implicated as a cause of heart disease, stroke, Alzheimer's disease, and cancer.

The average, 150-pound person requires about 55 to 80 grams of protein (about two to three ounces) daily. This is equivalent to about six to ten ounces of meat daily, if that were your only source of protein (and nearly all of us have many other sources).

To keep your animal protein intake down:

• Try limiting animal protein intake to no more than one serving (4 to 6 ounces) a day or less. This is roughly the size of the palm of your hand.

• Eat more vegetable proteins, including legumes (beans of all varieties), soy, whole grains, nuts, and seeds. These protein sources are less likely to raise homocysteine and are full of disease-fighting and healthful minerals, vitamins, and phytonutrients.

• Choose small fish (like sole or sardines) or egg whites as a high-quality protein source.

• Try soy products including tofu, edamame, soy milk, soy nuts, soy butter, and tempeh.

• When eating animal protein, choose lean sources such as poultry, leaner cuts of meat, or wild game such as elk and deer, which are low in saturated fat.

### Reduce Excess Alcohol

Although small amounts of alcohol (particularly red wine) may have health benefits, excessive alcohol has adverse effects. Besides leading to reduced mental acuity, alcohol also stimulates appetite and can lead to excess eating and weight gain.

Try to take a break from alcohol during the entire six-week ultraprevention plan period and watch what happens to your digestion, weight, sleep, sexual function, energy, and joint or muscle pains.

If you feel so good that you lose interest in drinking alcohol, terrific!

If you decide you absolutely can't avoid alcohol for six weeks, you might consider the possibility that you may have an alcohol issue.

If you can give it up for six weeks, but don't notice much change and you really miss a glass now and then, go back to drinking. But:

- Limit yourself to three to five drinks per week.
- Drink darker beers and red wine for the best health benefits.
- Try sulfite-free organic wine if you feel bad after drinking regular wine.

### Remove Vitamins and/or Medications with Fillers

Drug and vitamin manufacturers often include additives in their products for many reasons, particularly to make mass production possible and increase shelf life. They may also contain sweeteners and even extras like gluten and lactose (as in certain common thyroid medications) that can cause allergic reactions. Another common additive is aluminum (found in antacids, buffered aspirin, antidiarrheal medications, hemorrhoid medications, vaginal douches, and lipstick).

Find out what inactive ingredients are hidden in your medications and supplements. If you don't like what you see, try to find other forms or brands without those ingredients—health food stores are likely to carry them. (For more on vitamins, see page 280.)

## Remove Natural Food Carcinogens and Toxins

Some compounds found naturally in a variety of foods may be toxic and should be avoided. The most common examples are:

• Peanut butter, which can be contaminated with the carcinogen aflatoxin, which causes liver cancer. Aflatoxin is made by a mold called *Aspergillus flavus,* which grows in peanuts that have been stored improperly. The best way to avoid it is to keep your peanut butter refrigerated, and buy organic brands that screen for aflatoxin.

• Hydrazine, a known carcinogenic compound that is found in raw mushrooms. Mushrooms are just as good for you when cooked, so that's how we ask our patients to eat them.

• Charred (grilled) meats, which contain carcinogens known as *heterocyclic amines,* known to cause colorectal cancer.

• Acrylamide: Research on this toxin found in baked goods and fried starches has just been made available to the public, and indicates that we may need to reduce our intake of potato chips, french fries, and certain baked items.

### 2. ELIMINATE THE WASTE

Remove toxins from your environment and reduce the stress on your body's detoxification system.

## Clean Your Water

• Install a reverse osmosis system (a water purification system that you can buy through a dealer in the Yellow Pages) in your house for drinking water or for the whole system.

• If you don't have a filtration system for your whole house, attach a carbon filter (which you can get at any hardware store) to your shower and bath to reduce chlorine exposure.

• Consider bottled water when traveling away from home. You should also investigate the quality of your bottled water. For more information, read what water expert Dr. Mel Suffet, professor in the Environmental Science and Engineering Program at UCLA, has to say at www.ioe.ucla.edu/publications/report01/BottledWater.htm.

• Avoid drinking bottled water stored in a cloudy plastic container; the plastics leach into the water, especially when stored in hot conditions.

• Ask your local public health department for a reference lab in your area that assesses water quality—it's part of their job to oblige. Consider having your well or municipal water tested for levels of petrochemicals, heavy metals, and microorganisms.

## Clean Your Food

Eat organic food and animal products whenever possible to reduce your intake of petrochemical and pesticide residues, herbicides, fumigants, hormones, and antibiotics.

Toxic chemicals are dangerous and prevalent throughout our environment today. Consider the following:

• The Environmental Protection Agency (EPA) has found five of the most toxic chemicals in 100 percent of fat samples from cadaver surgical specimens, i.e., human corpses. These include OCDD, a dioxin; styrene; 1,4-dichlorobenzene; xylene; and ethylphenol. Presence in fat means they entered our bodies either through our food or water.

• Nine more chemicals were found in 91 to 98 percent of the cadavers. These include benzene, toluene, ethylbenzene, DDE (a breakdown product of DDT banned in the United States since 1972), and three dioxins.

• PCBs (polychlorinated biphenyls) were found in 83 percent.

• A recent Michigan study found DDT in over 70 percent of four-year-olds, probably received through breast milk.

• Almost 100 percent of beef is contaminated with DDT, as is 93 percent of processed cheese, hot dogs, bologna, turkey, and ice cream.

Toxic hormones are also dangerous. Dairy, and some beef products, often contain various growth hormones (bovine growth hormone or BGH, and bovine somatotropin, or BST) and residues of synthetic estrogens.

The dairy and beef industries use these hormones to increase milk production in dairy cattle and the weight of beef cattle. Even though DES (diethylstilbestrol), a synthetic estrogen, was known to cause cancer and birth defects in humans, until recently the beef industry used it to stimulate the growth of cows. Now the industry uses synthetic estrogen.

If all this weren't scary enough—be on the lookout for toxic metals, too. Government recommendations by the EPA, as well as several physicians' organizations, including the American College of Obstetrics and Gynecology (ACOG) and the American Academy of Pediatrics (AAP), all feel that children and pregnant women should avoid or limit their intake of tuna, swordfish, tilefish, king mackerel, and shark to minimize mercury exposure.

Fish from polluted lakes (such as pike, walleye, and bass), as well as large ocean fish, have also been found to contain unacceptably high levels of industrial toxins and heavy metals. (For more information on the EPA and FDA reports on fish and mercury, go to: www.epa.gov/mercury/fish.htm.)

Still another problem: antibiotics. According to the *New England Journal of Medicine* (October 18, 2001), "The Union of Concerned Scientists recently estimated that, each year, 24.6 million lbs (11.2 million kg) of antimicrobials are given to animals for nontherapeutic purposes and 2 million lbs (900,000 kg) are given for therapy; in contrast, 3 million lbs (1.3 million kg) are given to humans."

Researchers have found antibiotic-resistant bacteria in humans that originated from animal sources. Antibiotics given to animals are a major problem because they help create "superbacteria" that are highly resistant to the usual antibiotics. These bacteria have now been implicated in a range of human diseases, such as resistant salmonella from chicken.

Yet another issue is irradiated and genetically modified foods. New research suggests that irradiation of food produces previously nonexistent chemicals that have now been shown to have potentially carcinogenic effects. Irradiation of food also inactivates many of the important nutrients in food, specifically antioxidants (vitamins A, C, and E) and B-complex vitamins. No long-term studies of the health effects of irradiated food in humans have been conducted. Foods currently FDA-approved for radiation include wheat, wheat flour, fruits, vegetables, meats, poultry, teas, and spices.

Genetically modified foods are also now commonplace. These foods have been altered in the laboratory to produce genetically new strains that are resistant to pests or diseases. Soybeans, potatoes, and corn are some of the foods that have genetically modified strains. Again, no long-term human studies have been carried out to test the safety of these foods.

### How to choose your food

• Search out local markets for organic produce—whenever possible use certified organic fruits and vegetables. According to the FDA and the EPA, the twelve most contaminated foods are strawberries, peppers (red and green), spinach, cherries, peaches, cantaloupe (Mexican), celery, apples, apricots, green beans, grapes (Chilean), and cucumbers.

• Use eggs that are organic or are produced without antibiotics and hormones.

• Whenever possible, buy organic dairy products.

• Find local sources of free-range, organic meat, poultry, and other animal products.

• Limit your intake of large, predatory marine fish (such as tuna, swordfish, king mackerel, tilefish, shark, and halibut) to once a week.

- If you can't find completely organic animal products, next best are those raised without antibiotics or hormones.
- Beware of irradiated food. In the United States, irradiated food must be labeled with a seal.
- Genetically modified (GMO) foods do not require labeling. For resources on which food products may contain GMO ingredients, check the Greenpeace website at www.greenpeace.org.uk.

## Clean Your Air

Airborne exposures include far more than the usual dust, pollen, and molds. A major source is indoor air pollution—according to the EPA, indoor air pollution levels are often two to five times (and occasionally as much as one hundred times) higher than outdoor air pollution.

Here's how to clean the air around you:

### Purify your air

- HEPA/ULPA filters and ionizers can be helpful in reducing dust, molds, volatile organic compounds, and other sources of indoor air pollution.
- Clean and monitor your heating systems for release of carbon monoxide, the most common cause of death by poisoning in America.
- Use houseplants. Spider and banana plants can significantly reduce the formaldehyde levels in the air, and other live plants in your home or work environment act as natural air filters.

### Avoid excess exposure to airborne hazards

- Limit exposure to garden chemicals such as rotenone, Roundup (glyphosate), diazinon, and other pesticides and herbicides. Herbicides and pesticides should be used only sparingly in well-ventilated areas, ideally with protective respiratory masks such as chemical HEPA filters.

• Limit exposure to dry-cleaning solvents. If at all possible, consider hanging your dry-cleaned clothes outside to ventilate for a day before wearing.

• Car exhaust is toxic. Self-service gas stations may be cheaper, but spending time around them may be unhealthy.

• Reduce exposure to secondhand tobacco smoke as much as possible. Passive smoking has been linked to many respiratory disorders, as well as to cancer and heart disease.

• Do not microwave in Saran wrap or plastic wraps; use glass or ceramic containers when microwaving foods or storing hot food to reduce the leaching of the chemicals from plastics (phthalates) into your food.

• When entering your house, remove your shoes, especially if your house is carpeted, or you will track contaminants inside.

• Copiers, fax machines, and printers emit VOCs and should be used in well-ventilated spaces in your home office.

• Limit exposure to the following hazards: solvents, paints, paint removers, lacquers, adhesives, waxes and shellacs, fabric protectants (e.g., Scotchgard), nail polish (yes, nail polish), and polish remover.

• Avoid household petrochemicals by choosing natural alternatives (such as Citra-Solv orange-oil cleaner), or by providing adequate ventilation or air purification.

• Get more information about testing air for carbon monoxide and formaldehyde by calling the Consumer Products Safety Commission at (800) 638-2772.

• For information on how to measure the formaldehyde levels (as well as those of other common indoor air pollutants) in your house with home testing kits, go to www.aerias.org.

### Remove allergens

• Reduce exposure to dust mites as well as animal dander and hair by throwing out old carpets, pillows, and dust-collecting drapes.

• Keep animals out of the bedroom. Give them free rein in the rest of the house, but create at least one dander-free zone.

• Buy a dehumidifier if you live in a damp, warm climate to control mold and mold toxins. Shoot for a relative humidity of 35 to 40 percent.

• Air conditioners can be sources of mold. Make sure they are cleaned and maintained regularly.

• Consider antiallergenic mattress and pillow covers.

• Look for and remove toxic or highly allergenic molds in your house (basement, bathrooms, and so on).

• Throw out anything moldy, such as old carpets, blankets, strange old things in the basement, and science projects in the fridge.

• Use an ozone generator (available in mail-order catalogs) to kill molds, but only when no one is in the room. Wait an hour after use before entering the space.

## Reduce Heavy Metal Exposure

### Reduce lead exposure

The most common source of lead is general household dust, particularly in older buildings or neighborhoods. Older buildings (built prior to 1950) often have layers of lead paint, which can cause significant exposure if the paint is chipping or sanded off. Toddlers can absorb toxins from lead through playing in dirt. Additional unsuspected sources of lead can include:

• Calcium supplement tablets. Significant amounts of lead have been measured in name-brand calcium carbonate supplements from different sources, including oyster shells, bonemeal, and dolomite. Look for calcium supplements that are labeled "lead-free" or "virtually lead-free."

• Antacids containing calcium.

• Vinyl miniblinds, when manufactured before 1996, can produce lead dust as they deteriorate.

• Homes with lead pipes or copper pipes with lead solder.

• Car batteries, fishing sinkers, bullets, lead solder, and stained glass.

### Reduce mercury exposure

Limit your intake of swordfish, tuna, tilefish, shark, and other large carnivorous fish. Additional sources of mercury include:

• Broken thermometers or blood pressure cuffs
• Silver (amalgam) dental fillings
• Antiseptics containing mercurochrome
• Contact lens solutions containing thimerosal (mercury)
• Vaccines containing thimerosal
• Old (pre-1990) latex paint

### Reduce cadmium exposure

Cadmium is a toxic metal that damages the lungs when inhaled or the stomach when swallowed. Long-term exposure to cadmium is also thought to cause kidney disease and osteoporosis, as well as lung and prostate cancer. You can reduce your cadmium exposure by:

• Eliminating your exposure to tobacco smoke—a pack of cigarettes contains about 20 mcg of cadmium, or 1 mcg per cigarette.

• Avoiding exposure to fertilizers.

• Reducing intake of coffee, which also contains cadmium.

### Reduce arsenic exposure

Arsenic is a poisonous metal with many adverse health effects including cancer of the lung, kidney, bladder, and liver, as well as nerve injury, hearing loss, diabetes, and adverse effects on the cardiovascular system. Arsenic can be a contaminant in drinking water as well as bottled water. Another important source of arsenic exposure is treated wood (pressure-treated wood resists molds and weathering due to its arsenic content).

Your doctor can test your arsenic level if you are concerned. You can also talk to your local Department of Public Works about the arsenic levels in your water. And home test kits and test strips are available at stores such as Home Depot for some heavy metals. For more information on toxins in the home, go to www.epa.gov.

### Minimize Radiation Exposure

Radiation can have significant harmful health effects, particularly as a cause of cancer. The stronger the radiation, the higher the risk. Radiation exposure comes from a variety of sources of varying strengths:

#### Radon gas

Radon is a naturally occurring radioactive gas that can seep into homes through cracks in the foundation and become trapped due to tight insulation. The EPA has set safe limits for radon levels in homes at 4 pCi/L (or picocuries per liter). Currently, about one in fifteen homes in the United States exceeds this limit. You can order an inexpensive kit to test your home from many local government and community organizations. For more information, contact the National Radon Safety Board at www.nrsb.org.

#### Air travel

Flying exposes you to significant amounts of ionizing radiation. The air is thinner high above the earth, offering less protection from radiation. If possible, reduce plane trips—the International Commission on Radiation Protection sets the recommended limit at 5 millisieverts (500 millirems) of radiation a year. Ten trips a year can mean about 3 millisieverts (300 millirems) of exposure.

### Sunshine

Use sunscreen whenever you plan to be outdoors in the sun (it wards off wrinkles, too). Also use UV-protection sunglasses to prevent cataracts.

### Electromagnetic fields from cell phones

Cell phones may cause potentially adverse health effects, although adequate research has not yet been done. It appears that cell phones can cause increases in blood pressure and constriction of blood vessels, according to a 1998 report in *The Lancet* (June 20, 1998). Hands-free speakerphone setups for cell phones in cars reduce your exposure to electromagnetic radiation.

### Computers

If you spend a lot of time in front of a CRT computer screen, invest in a screen protector that blocks some of the radiation exposure. Also, sit farther away from your computer screen. LCD (flat-panel) monitors generate less radiation than standard cathode screens.

### Power lines

There has been much public discussion about the effect of living near power lines, and a possible increase in cancer rates, but we are not aware of any definitive study on the subject.

### 3. REMOVE THE RUST

Clear your body of excess free radicals.

Many factors contribute to aging and disease, but one of the most important of all is what we call rust, or oxidative stress. You name it: heart disease, Alzheimer's, Parkinson's, arthritis, diabetes, kidney disease, macular degeneration, and skin wrinkles—these are all manifestations of unchecked rust.

The culprits who do the damage are free radicals, which, as discussed, are highly reactive oxygen molecules that damage tissues they come into contact with in precisely the same way that oxygen can cause metal to rust and apples to turn brown when exposed to air. Free radicals are a normal part of our body's chemistry, but when the production of free radicals exceeds our body's ability to absorb them, damage to our cells begins.

There are two ways to reduce this damage. First, limit the body's production of free radicals. Second, strengthen and support your body's antioxidant system.

## Diet

### Reduce excess calories in your diet
The first foods to cut down on or eliminate are those with low nutrient-to-calorie ratios (NCR). Low-NCR foods have a lot of calories relative to their nutrient content, and so these foods increase the amount of oxidative stress, or rust, our bodies are exposed to. The highest NCR foods are vegetables and fruits. You can imagine where colas and doughnuts fit on this scale! (For more on high- and low-NCR foods, see page 274.)

### Increase your intake of antioxidant-rich foods
These foods are usually easy to spot because they are often so colorful. Look for fruits and vegetables containing antioxidants such as carotenes, luteins, lycopenes, xanthines, xeanthins, and proantho-cyanidins, found in carrots, blueberries, yams, tomatoes, and peppers.

### Reduce or eliminate sugar from your diet
Sugar is one of the best examples of a low-NCR food: pure calories providing no other nutrition. This leads to the production of excess free radicals. Sugar also taxes our antioxidant system because it does not provide any antioxidants—it only uses them up.

### *Remove rancid fats from your diet*

Oil that has turned rancid in nuts, vegetable oils, or animal fats is a source of carcinogens and oxidative stress. Consider keeping nuts and vegetable oils in the refrigerator (except olive oil, which will solidify in the fridge).

## Environment

### *Eliminate environmental sources of oxidative stress*

You know tobacco smoke (first- or secondhand) is bad. Tobacco smoke released from burning (oxidized) tobacco pours free radicals directly into your circulation through the lungs. No wonder that smoking causes aging, wrinkles, cancer, heart attack, and stroke.

Unnecessary medications, even over-the-counter ones such as Tylenol or Motrin that are largely considered safe, can add to oxidative stress, and liver and kidney damage when taken in excessive amounts.

Also look out for pesticides and other environmental petrochemicals, solvents, heavy metals, carbon monoxide, and nitrogen dioxide.

## Lifestyle

### *Exercise*

There's a reason exercise is so heavily recommended. It's good for you! Exercise regularly—but not to excess. Regular exercise reduces oxidative stress, but overexercising, like overeating, taxes the body's equilibrium and leads to increased oxidative stress. This may explain why marathon runners often get sick or come down with infections after a race—their immune systems are suppressed because of increased oxidative stress.

*Sleep*

Improve your sleep habits. Maintaining regular and adequate duration of sleeping, waking, and eating is key for balance. If the body's
circadian rhythms and hormonal patterns are out of kilter, increased
oxidative stress can result.

*Reduce stress*

We know this is easy to say, but taking action to reduce stress can have
immeasurable health benefits and can reduce rust. This may mean
practicing a relaxation technique on a regular basis, or reexamining
your priorities. Since everyone reacts to stress differently, it's not the
amount of stress that's important, but rather how you react to it.

For more on these three subjects, and other lifestyle issues, see
Step Three.

## 4. COOL THE HEAT
Free your body of inflammation.

Inflammation, or what we call heat, is a normal response of our
immune system. When we get an infection, our immune system
creates an inflammatory reaction, which serves to recruit more
"fighting" cells to an area of concern; it's one way our immune system calls for backup when confronting a potential problem.

But once the process of inflammation is initiated, it's hard to
quiet down. Inflammation then becomes a smoldering fire that
causes damage to tissues.

There are just a few primary causes of inflammation:

• Infections—these can be caused by bacteria, viruses, yeasts and
molds, parasites, and other unusual organisms. Common locations
of unsuspected infections include: teeth, sinuses, gut (gastrointestinal tract), and reproductive tract—prostate, cervix, and so on.
   • Environmental and food allergies
   • Weight gain and being overweight

- Insulin resistance (see page 261)
- Autoimmune conditions such as arthritis, colitis, and lupus
- Injuries

If the source of inflammation is identified, it should be targeted and eliminated. If the source of inflammation is unknown, a general anti-inflammatory approach is recommended, including following an anti-inflammatory diet and taking supplements. Here are ways to cool the heat of inflammation:

## Eliminate Suspected and Unsuspected Sources of Infection

### Teeth

Gum (periodontal) disease can harbor smoldering infections, as can bad cavities, old root canals, implants, and bridges. Follow these steps to reduce those sources of inflammation:

- See your dentist and/or periodontist regularly for preventive maintenance.
- Floss your teeth daily.
- Brush regularly.
- Consider an ultrasonic brush and water pick for daily use to improve plaque removal.

### Sinuses

Sinus infections can be reduced by promoting proper drainage of the mucus in the sinuses, as well as by avoiding allergens that make the membranes lining the sinuses swell and become congested, and then blocked, which leads to infection. Follow these steps to reduce sinus infections:

- Stay well hydrated. Drink plenty of water, which thins sinus mucus and promotes drainage.

• Drink hot beverages.

• Exercise and indulge in saunas and steam to increase sweating.

• Try regular sinus irrigation, using a saltwater solution (a good device for this is RinoFlow—www.entdr.com/rinoflow.html).

• Try to avoid drying decongestants, antihistamines, and over-the-counter nasal sprays. These provide temporary relief, but are often followed by a rebound congestion that can be very severe.

### Gastrointestinal tract

A number of organisms can cause infections in the gastrointestinal tract and create continued inflammation. These are most often acquired by eating contaminated food, but imbalances in the ecology of the intestinal tract may also occur as a result of antibiotic use, stress, or improper diet. Here are some steps to reduce gastrointestinal infections:

• Take antibiotics only when necessary—most colds, upper respiratory infections, and even sinus infections do not require antibiotics. (If you must take an antibiotic, supplement it with acidophilus.)

• Maintain a high-soluble-fiber diet; this encourages and promotes the health of beneficial bacteria in the gut, such as acidophilus and bifidobacteria.

• Avoid foods you may be sensitive or allergic to. The most common food allergies include dairy, wheat (gluten), soy, nuts, eggs, and shellfish.

• All produce should be carefully washed before eating, especially nondomestic fruits and berries, which can harbor organisms such as cyclospora.

• Identify and treat ecological imbalances in the gut. Overgrowth of undesirable bacteria and yeasts often occurs as a result of antibiotic use, stress, or poor diet. Restoring the ecological balance of gut microorganisms is an important part of cooling the heat. The objective is to replace undesirable microbes with beneficial, "symbiotic" bacteria (bacteria that are helpful to us, as we are to them) such as acidophilus, bifidobacteria, and the friendly forms of *E. coli*. Take these as well as more fiber and less sugar. Some herbs and their extracts, too, may be helpful, such as oil of oregano, garlic, citrus seed extract, berberine, plant tannins, undecylenate, and caprylic acid.

• Intestinal parasites are not uncommon and also should be identified and treated. A stool sample sent to an experienced lab can identify most intestinal parasites. Treatment often requires medications such as Flagyl, Humatin, or Yodoxin, although some herbals, such as artemisia, oil of oregano, and berberine, may also be helpful. Another common infection is caused by *Helicobacter pylori,* which causes stomach ulcers and heartburn and can eventually lead to stomach cancer. This infection is curable with the right combination of antibiotics.

• When restoring ecological balance in the gut, it's best to work with an experienced practitioner. Visit our website at www.ultraprevention.com for more information.

### Reproductive tract

The reproductive tract is particularly vulnerable to infections because of sexual contact, and these infections can be a source of ongoing inflammation. Check with your doctor to rule out infections such as:

• Bacterial vaginitis: This may cause a discharge, itching, or discomfort.

• Cervicitis: Infections of the cervix are common, particularly with viruses such as HPV, the human papilloma virus. This infection also affects men, and is thought to occur in up to 75 percent of sexually active women. It causes genital warts and cervical cancer.

• Prostatitis: A chronic, smoldering infection in the prostate gland, it is a common male affliction, affecting up to 35 percent of men over age 50. Symptoms include difficulty urinating, low back pain, testicular pain, or painful ejaculation.

## Control Your Allergies

Allergies are reactions not just to airborne substances like dust, pollen, and mold but to foods as well. Food allergies are much more common than most people realize and can be a source of ongoing stimulation and activation of the immune system, causing inflammation.

Here are steps we recommend to reduce sources of allergens:

For six weeks, try to eliminate the top three sources of allergies from your diet—dairy, wheat and gluten, and eggs. You may notice the following significant changes:

- Less abdominal bloating and gas
- More energy
- More regular bowel habits
- Less heartburn and indigestion
- Clearer sinuses and better breathing
- Fewer joint pains and stiffness
- Clearer skin

Remove sources of common environmental allergies such as:

- Dust
- Mold
- Pet hair and dander

## Achieve and Maintain a Healthy Weight

Simply being overweight can cause low-grade chronic inflammation. The severity of this inflammation can be measured by your doctor with a C-reactive protein blood test (see page 205). If you're overweight and have any sign of inflammation, then we strongly suggest achieving and maintaining a healthy weight.

We could write an entire book on this subject, but here are some basic suggestions:

- Eat primarily high-NCR foods.
- Increase fiber in your diet through such sources as legumes, nuts, and whole cereals—aim for 30 grams of fiber daily or more (or at least 15 grams of fiber for every 1,000 calories you eat).
- Limit or eliminate sugar, refined grains, and starchy carbohydrates from your diet—these increase appetite and lead to weight gain.
- Try aerobic exercise (at least four times a week) and strength training (three times a week).

### Combat Insulin Resistance

If you're one of the more than 30 percent of Americans with insulin resistance, you must address this problem through diet, exercise, and certain supplements.

The easiest test for insulin resistance is the waist/hip measurement. Here you simply measure your waist around your belly button and then measure the widest point of your hips, and divide the former measurement by the latter. If the result is more than 0.8 (for women) or 0.9 (for men), you may be insulin resistant. You can also ask your doctor for a blood test.

Insulin resistance has a direct effect in causing inflammation. To combat and reduce insulin resistance, follow our guidelines for the treatment of insulin resistance syndrome (see page 264).

### Target Inflammatory Conditions and Injuries

Although anti-inflammatory medications such as ibuprofen can help reduce some of the symptoms as well as some of the complications of inflammation, we prefer a dietary and nutritional approach.

Try eating fewer of the foods that trigger or aggravate inflammation, while increasing foods that reduce it.

Here are some guidelines:

• Eliminate or reduce your intake of red meats, egg yolks, and shellfish. These foods are high in a fat known as arachidonic acid, which initiates the inflammatory process.

• Supplement your diet with healthy sources of the essential omega-3 fatty acids EPA and ALA by increasing your intake of fish and fish oils, ground flaxseed or flax oil, pumpkin seeds, walnuts, and soybeans.

• Increase your intake of anti-inflammatory foods and spices such as turmeric (and its derivative curcumin), ginger, garlic, onions, cayenne, rosemary, citrus fruits, and parsley.

• Increase your fiber intake from foods such as whole grains, fruits and vegetables, nuts, seeds, and legumes.

## 5. END THE BURNOUT
Feel energized by maximizing your metabolism.

Ultimately, metabolism is simply the body's process of using the oxygen we breathe and the food we eat to make the energy we need to maintain all bodily functions. As you will recall from Part II, the place where we create this energy (in the form of the high-energy chemical ATP) is in our mitochondria.

Many things can go wrong during the formation of ATP that can impair our metabolism, make it run less efficiently, or almost shut it down.

Burnout, or impaired metabolism, results in loss of cellular function as well as physical energy. This energy crisis means more than just feeling tired. The loss of energy on a cellular basis is often the first step of dysfunction that leads to many diseases, from heart and liver failure to Parkinson's and Alzheimer's.

There are many causes of burnout. These include mitochondrial malfunction, insulin resistance, thyroid dysfunction, oxidative stress, and other hormonal imbalances.

## Avoid Mitochondrial Malfunction

Fatigue and pain are the most common complaints patients bring to their doctors. At their core, both are related to damaged or poorly functioning mitochondria. Mitochondria, as you may recall, are the tiny power plants of our cells; they produce the energy our cells need by converting food to ATP, the basic currency of energy in our bodies. A cell that can't make enough energy is in big trouble.

The cascade of events that leads to cell death goes something like this: Cellular repair stops, toxins accumulate, free radicals run rampant, and the cell dies. This cascade begins with mitochondrial malfunction.

Mitochondria are susceptible to injury from a number of causes. Here are some causes of mitochondrial malfunction and how to remove them:

### Overeating

Consuming too many calories puts undue strain on the mitochondria by asking them to process more calories than they're able to. Remember to choose foods with a high NCR. If you'd like to increase your calorie intake, then you should first increase the number of mitochondria you have through aerobic exercise (see over).

### Heavy metal exposure

Heavy metals such as mercury, lead, arsenic, and cadmium have a toxic effect on mitochondria. Reduce food and environmental sources of heavy metal exposure. This means reducing your intake of large predatory marine fish (tuna, swordfish, et cetera).

### Undernutrition

A lack of vitamins and minerals may deplete levels of nutrients essential for optimal mitochondrial function.

### Stress

Practicing stress reduction techniques on a regular basis can help your mitochondria stay healthy.

### Lack of exercise

Probably the best way to keep your mitochondria healthy is to engage in regular aerobic exercise. Aerobic exercise prompts our bodies to manufacture new, young, and healthy mitochondria. We recommend thirty minutes of aerobic exercise four days per week.

### Medication toxicity

Some medications can interfere with mitochondrial function and energy production, such as HIV drugs (protease inhibitors), statins (cholesterol-lowering drugs), cancer chemotherapy drugs, some anticonvulsants (anti-epilepsy drugs) such as Depakote, and tetracycline (an antibiotic). Ask your doctor about any side effects you may be experiencing while taking medications.

### Rust

Rust (or oxidative stress) also affects our delicate mitochondria. See "Remove the Rust," page 253.

## Target Insulin Resistance

Insulin resistance occurs when the body loses its responsiveness to the hormone insulin. This condition is aggravated and accentuated when there is an improper diet, or when lifestyle disorders such as stress, insomnia, lack of exercise, or substance abuse are present. Insulin resistance causes weight gain (particularly around the middle of the body), fatigue, mental fogginess, low HDL, and eventually high blood pressure, cardiovascular disease, and at times even dementia and cancer.

To minimize the effects of insulin resistance, follow these guidelines:

### Eliminate the White Menace

As discussed, white foods are often high in sugar or can be converted quickly into sugar in our bodies, and this should be avoided if you are insulin resistant. These include foods such as white flour, white pasta, white rice, white bread, white potatoes, cereals, and sugar itself.

### Increase your fiber intake

Fiber slows down the body's absorption of sugar. Aim for at least thirty grams of fiber daily in your diet. High-fiber sources include fruits and vegetables, beans, nuts and seeds, and whole grains.

### Reduce stress

Here it is again, that dreaded stress. One of the harmful effects of stress is to raise your body's level of cortisol, a hormone from the adrenal glands that directly aggravates insulin resistance. Don't do stress!

### Get moving

Exercise has a powerful and direct effect on restoring the body's sensitivity to insulin. Exercise works better than any medication and is a necessary ingredient in the recipe to overcome insulin resistance.

### Don't light the midnight oil

Restful, restorative sleep also helps to improve insulin resistance by lowering cortisol levels. If you're burning both ends of the candle, you're more prone to insulin resistance and its harmful effects.

## ,ort the Thyroid

thyroid gland (a butterfly-shaped gland in the neck on either side of the voice box, or larynx) is an important organ that can be thought of as the body's thermostat. The thyroid controls a multitude of bodily functions, including our body temperature, heart rate, metabolic rate, cholesterol levels, hair, skin and nail growth, bowel function, and dozens of other functions.

To support the thyroid, we need to eliminate causes of thyroid dysfunction, which include:

### Selenium deficiency

Selenium is a necessary mineral for proper thyroid function. Thyroid disease is epidemic in areas of the world where selenium levels in the soil and therefore in vegetables is low. In America, selenium deficiency can be found in the coastal Northwest (Washington, Oregon, northern California), the Northeast (New England), parts of the Midwest (Ohio, Indiana, Iowa), and Florida. Low selenium causes hypothyroidism, or an underactive thyroid. The recommended daily allowance for selenium is 55 to 70 mcg/day, but research suggests that intakes of 200 mcg/day may also protect against cancer of the lung, colon, prostate, and some (nonmelanoma) skin cancers. High amounts of selenium can cause side effects, so don't take more than 400 mcg/day. Good sources of selenium include Brazil nuts, turkey and chicken, eggs, brown rice, and walnuts—but remember that if you are eating a lot of these foods, you should lower the amount of your selenium supplements accordingly.

### Iodine deficiency

Iodine is an integral part of the thyroid's effective function. Iodine deficiency, which can cause a goiter (an enlargement of the thyroid gland), is less common since iodine was added to table salt in 1924. The recommended intake of iodine to prevent deficiency is between

150 and 200 mcg/day for adults (less for children). Dietary sources include fish (which can be quite high in iodine, around 500 mcg in six ounces of marine fish), iodized salt, kelp, and shellfish. Few of us need supplementation, as Western diets usually have sufficient iodine content.

### Hormone use

Women taking hormones, either in the form of a birth control pill or as menopausal hormone therapy, may have alterations in thyroid function that may require a change in treatment. See www.ultraprevention.com to learn more about getting a blood test.

### Environmental toxins

Avoid chemicals and mercury—small amounts of these potent hormone disruptors can significantly affect the thyroid and other endocrine organs (sex organs and adrenal glands).

### Essential fatty acid deficiency

Essential fats are important in helping thyroid hormones do their work at the cell membrane.

### Adrenal disfunction

Low thyroid function and low adrenal function can each make the other condition worse. Be sure to treat and deal with adrenal dysfunction when it occurs.

### Gluten allergy

This results in celiac disease, and may be present if the thyroid is malfunctioning.

# STEP TWO: REPAIR—THE SECOND TWO WEEKS

**GOALS:**
1. Repair the Digestive System and Optimize Nutrition
2. Repair and Enhance Detoxification
3. Repair the Rust: Oil the Oxidative Stress System
4. Repair Immune Function and Reduce Inflammation
5. Repair Metabolism

**1. Repair the Digestive System and Optimize Nutrition**
In some ways our digestive system is similar to a complex ecosystem like a rain forest, inhabited by a multitude of differing flora. And like a rain forest, our digestive system is very susceptible to influences that can have a ripple effect throughout the entire works.

The forces that disturb that equilibrium are rampant in our culture: poor diet, food allergens, toxic food additives, infections, alcohol, medications (especially antibiotics), anti-inflammatories and acid-blocking drugs, various illnesses, and stress.

The importance of a healthy digestive system for overall health and vitality cannot be overstated. Research has connected digestive problems to symptoms and diseases far outside the gut, including allergies, asthma, eczema, arthritis, brain diseases, autism, fibromyalgia, and chronic fatigue.

By repairing the digestive system first, we can ensure that the nutrients we consume will be properly absorbed so that we can make use of these critical building blocks of health.

After we repair the digestive system, we optimize nutrition.

Here is a strategy for repairing damage to the digestive tract from a lifetime of insults.

### Try an Elimination Diet

Many common ailments will resolve with a brief (two- to six-week) trial of an elimination diet. Such a diet can give even those without particular symptoms or obvious allergies a chance to rest the digestive tract and the immune system, allowing for deep healing and repair.

During this elimination phase, the following foods should be avoided:

- Wheat and gluten-containing foods
- Dairy products
- Eggs
- Sugar and refined grains
- Corn
- Peanuts
- Caffeine
- Processed or packaged foods
- Alcohol

Why these foods? They include the most common food allergens (which can trigger inflammation and irritation of the intestinal lining), rust-causing foods (sugar and refined grains), and foods that can impair metabolism or encourage sludge (malnutrition).

Now you're thinking . . . what *can* I eat? During this elimination phase you should concentrate on eating a diet composed of organic, high-fiber, fresh, unprocessed food, such as:

- Colorful vegetables and fruits
- Beans

• Whole grains (except those containing gluten: wheat, oats, rye, barley, spelt, kamut)
  • Omega-3 fatty acids (flaxseed and wild fish)
  • Olive oil
  • Lean animal protein (including fish)
  • Nuts and seeds

These foods, the foundation of a lifelong ultraprevention diet, are high in vitamins, minerals, antioxidants, anti-inflammatory compounds, fiber, and essential fatty acids. These foundation foods also eliminate the many triggers of chronic illness: saturated fat and trans fats, sugar, empty calories, hormones, antibiotics, and toxic food additives that are everyday fare for most Americans.

## Take Probiotics

Many things can deplete or destroy our normal healthy bacteria. These include a poor diet, alcohol, antibiotics, acid-blocking drugs, stress, and infections. Probiotic supplements are simply capsules of purified beneficial bacteria. Although yogurt is fine, it cannot provide adequate quantities of bacteria by itself.

For six weeks, replace the healthy bacteria as follows:

• Look for reputable, refrigerated brands of mixed flora, including healthy bacteria such as *Lactobacillus acidophilus*, *Lactobacillus rhamnosis,* and/or *Bifidobacteria bifidum*. All of these can be found at any good health store.
• Take a supplement that provides, per its label, five to ten billion organisms a day on an empty stomach in divided doses (twice a day).
• Refrigerate probiotics in airtight storage containers.

## Increase Fiber Intake

Our healthy bacteria require fiber as their principle source of food. By eating fiber, we make sure that the probiotic supplements we take actually "stick" and lead to the growth of healthy bacterial colonies in our gastrointestinal tract. Fiber also promotes waste elimination, fights colon cancer, lowers cholesterol, and regulates proper hormone balance.

The average American consumes only about 8 grams of fiber a day. Instead, aim for 25 to 50 grams every day, with a mixture of soluble and insoluble fibers. Our guidelines recommend at least 15 grams of fiber for every 1,000 calories you eat.

To increase fiber intake:

• Make flaxseed a part of your everyday diet: Try one to two tablespoons a day of ground flaxseed. You can buy preground organic flaxseed or grind your own (and keep it refrigerated). Add it to salads, sprinkle it over vegetables, mix it in unsweetened organic applesauce, or eat it plain.

• Eat beans (and all forms of legumes).

• Load up on vegetables—with almost no calories, high levels of antioxidants and protective phytochemicals, these excellent fiber sources should be heaped on your plate daily.

• Eat whole grains such as brown rice or quinoa.

• Include a few servings of low-sugar fruits in your daily diet (berries have the highest content of fiber and other protective phytochemicals).

• Add one or two handfuls of nuts, such as almonds, walnuts, pecans, or hazelnuts, to your diet every day.

• Consider a good fiber supplement that contains soluble and insoluble fibers. Or think about taking unsweetened psyllium seed husks—take one or two tablespoons a day, and be sure to wash it down with plenty of water.

• Start slowly. Switching abruptly to a high-fiber diet can cause gas and bloating. Increase intake slowly until you reach your goal of 25 to 50 grams per day.

## Try Digestive Enzymes and Digestive Bitters

Poor digestion is not an uncommon problem. Symptoms may include gas, bloating, or an excessive feeling of fullness after meals. Using supplemental digestive enzymes may be helpful. Most health food stores carry a variety of different digestive enzymes, which can be taken at the beginning of each meal to help support complete digestion.

Or you could try digestive bitters. Swedish bitters or other aperitifs stimulate digestive function, including production of enzymes and stomach acid. Consider taking some before each meal per the manufacturer's instructions. Herbal bitters that include gentian and artichoke, cardamom, fennel, ginger, and dandelion are also available in more concentrated forms that can be added to water and taken as an elixir before meals.

---

### CONFUSED ABOUT EGGS?

If so, you're not alone. It's hard to keep up with egg research. In general, we like eggs, especially the new omega eggs (which have been created to be high in omega-3 fats, accomplished by feeding the chickens themselves more omega-3s).

There are two major concerns with eggs:
1. Eggs are a fairly common food allergen, so if you're allergic to eggs it's best to avoid them.
2. Egg yolks contain arachidonic acid, one of the fats that leads to inflammation. So egg yolks should generally be avoided if you have any inflammatory condition (but egg whites would still be fine in this situation).

---

## Fix Your Eating Habits

Often *how* we eat is just as important as *what* we eat. If we are stressed, eat too quickly, eat too much at one time, or eat too late at night, our digestion is affected. By following a few simple guide-lines, you can improve your digestion immeasurably and you might even lose weight or get rid of that nagging indigestion or irritable bowel syndrome.

• Chew each mouthful 25 to 50 times—or at least try! This re-leases EGF—epithelial growth factor—which is needed for repair and healing of the digestive lining.

• Eat slowly and don't do anything else while eating.

• Take pleasure in meals by taking the time to enjoy them with friends or family, or by creating simple mealtime rituals such as a blessing, lighting of candles, or anything else resulting in a soothing environment.

• Eat smaller, more frequent meals.

• Mix it up by including carbohydrates, fat, protein, and fiber in each meal.

• Don't eat anything for three hours before bedtime.

• Breathe! Try taking five deep breaths before you eat—breathe in for five seconds and out for five seconds, and do this five times. You will be amazed at how easy and yet how powerful such a sim-ple exercise can be.

## Follow the Ultraprevention Diet

As mentioned, it's quite possible to be both overweight and mal-nourished (what we call overconsumptive-undernourished) at the same time. If you're eating a great deal of food, but none of it is nutritious, you've got a combination that's a prescription for dis-ease.

With this in mind, we offer an ultrapreventative diet to help you eat as healthily as possible. While different people with different body types and genetic predispositions need different diets, our guidelines provide a sensible foundation for a lifetime of sound and intelligent eating that can help defeat the five forces of illness.

In general, we can separate foods into high-, medium-, or low-quality categories based on their NCR, or nutrient-to-calorie ratio. Our objective is to eat mostly high-NCR foods and few low-NCR foods.

Picture a food pyramid with three levels. The largest level contains the high-NCR foods, the middle level contains the medium-NCR foods, and the top, or smallest, level contains the low-NCR foods. Through this simple concept a healthy eating pattern can be developed that is not a diet, but a program that enriches your metabolism, supports your immune system, aids detoxification, and reduces inflammation and oxidative stress while correcting malnutrition.

Because we're all different, some of us may need more fat, or less fat, or may have higher protein needs, or not tolerate starchy carbohydrates. The best barometer of what you need is how you feel. When you eat properly for your constitution and metabolism, you should feel great—even after just six weeks. Pay attention to how the food you eat makes you feel and experiment with different amounts of different categories of nutrients. You are your own best judge of what works for you.

When you eat properly for your body, your weight will become normal, your energy will improve, and often many seemingly unrelated physical complaints will disappear.

### High-NCR Foods
Eat at least 8 to 10 servings a day (1 serving = ½ cup) of each.

### 1. Vegetables
Vegetables should be organic and fresh whenever possible.
The best are:
• Cruciferous vegetables (broccoli, brussels sprouts, cauliflower, kohlrabi, cabbage)

- Dark green leafy vegetables (escarole, Swiss chard, collard greens, kale, spinach, and dandelion, mustard, or beet greens)
- Colorful vegetables:
    Red: tomatoes, chili peppers, red bell peppers
    Green: green beans, asparagus, green peppers, okra, snow peas, zucchini
    Yellow: yellow squash, fresh corn
    Purple: eggplant, beets
    White (yes, we know white has no color, but bear with us): mushrooms, sprouts, water chestnuts, bamboo shoots, lotus root, burdock root

Plus:

- Lettuce/mixed greens—arugula, romaine, red and green leaf, endive, radicchio, chicory, watercress
- Sea vegetables—wakame, kombu, nori, arame, hijiki
- Allium vegetables—garlic, onions, shallots, leeks, scallions

## 2. Fruit

Focus on fresh, organic fruits with low glycemic levels; these include berries (blueberries, raspberries, blackberries), apples, pears, kiwis, mangoes, citrus, peaches, apricots, nectarines, and plums.

## 3. Plant proteins

- Red, green, or French lentils; green or yellow split peas
- Beans: kidney, navy, lima, mung, pinto, black, and garbanzo (chickpeas)
- Soy foods (tofu, tempeh, soy milk, soy yogurt, soy nuts, edamame)

**Medium-NCR Foods**
Eat 4 to 5 servings a day.

### 1. Animal proteins

- Free-range, organic, or DHA (omega-3) eggs
- Low-fat or nonfat organic yogurt
- Wild game, including elk and deer
- Wild fish (not farm raised, which are processed with antibiotics and medications), including wild salmon, arctic char, halibut, sea bass, sardines, herring, trout, and sole
- Lean poultry (white meat) from free-range chicken, turkey, Cornish game hen
- Lean red meats such as roast beef and lamb

### 2. Healthful oils

- Organic flaxseed oil
- Organic borage oil
- Organic extra virgin olive oil
- Small amounts of cold-pressed or expeller-pressed polyunsaturated oils, including sesame, walnut, and almond

---

### LEARN WHAT A PORTION REALLY IS

- ½ cup is the general serving size—this is about equal to a tennis ball.
- 3 ounces is the size of an animal protein serving (about the size of your palm). For other proteins: 2 eggs, 8 ounces or 1 cup of tofu, ½ cup of legumes.
- Vegetables: One serving = ½ cup.
- Nuts and seeds: One serving = 10 to 12 nuts or 1 tablespoon of nut butter.
- Cooked grains: One serving = ½ cup.
- Whole grain bread: One serving = 1 slice.
- Dairy: One serving = 6 ounces of yogurt.
- Oil: One serving = 1 tablespoon of oil (olive or flax, etc.), 8 to 10 olives, or ⅛ of an avocado.

---

### 3. Nuts and seeds

Organic almonds, hazelnuts, walnuts, pecans, Brazil nuts, cashews, pistachios, sunflower seeds, pumpkin seeds, sesame seeds, and flaxseed, as well as organic nut butters (almond, macadamia, cashew, sunflower, soy)

### 4. Whole grains

• Brown rice, wild rice, quinoa, millet, buckwheat, barley, steel-cut oats, rye, spelt, kamut, amaranth
• Whole grain breads and whole grain pastas

### 5. Fruits and vegetables

• Starchy vegetables, root vegetables such as sweet potatoes, winter squashes, turnips, rutabagas, carrots, parsnips
• Avocados
• Olives
• Moderate amounts of higher-glycemic fruits, including pineapples, bananas, grapes, melons

### Low-NCR Foods

Avoid these whenever possible.

### 1. Low-NCR carbohydrates

• White flour
• White bread
• White potatoes
• White rice
• Cereals
• Alcohol
• White sugar
• All other forms of sugar—evaporated cane sugar, honey, molasses, Sucanat, maple syrup, barley malt, brown rice syrup, high-fructose corn syrup—and all foods containing them

- Popcorn
- Rice cakes

## 2. Low-NCR Fats and Oils

- Trans or hydrogenated fats, such as margarine and shortening
- Refined polyunsaturated oils, such as corn, sunflower, or safflower
- Saturated fat from animal sources (beef, pork, lamb, chicken, dairy products—but keep in mind that you can eat low-fat or non-fat dairy products)
- Cocoa butter
- Butter
- Tropical oils, including palm and coconut oil

## 3. Junk foods

- Sodas
- Fast food
- Fried food (especially breaded fried foods)
- Desserts
- Snack foods

## Cooking with Condiments

Spices do more than add wonderful flavors to your meals—they are also full of healing properties. Here are some to keep in mind when you prepare your next meal:

- Turmeric can significantly reduce inflammation.
- Ginger is an antioxidant, a digestive aid, and reduces inflammation.
- Rosemary enhances detoxification and also reduces inflammation.
- Sage can increase the flow of bile and liver detoxification.

• Garlic has abundant healing properties—it thins the blood, reduces blood pressure, lowers cholesterol, improves immunity, fights microbes, and may protect against cancer.

• Oregano has twelve antibiotic, antifungal, antiviral, and anti-parasitic compounds.

• Cinnamon has antifungal properties.

• Burdock increases urine and sweat production.

## Maximize Methylation

A key objective in correcting malnutrition is maximizing methylation. Methylation is a crucial step for our bodies in the process of repairing our DNA, controlling which of our genes are turned on or off, and producing proteins.

Here's how to maximize methylation:

• Monitor and maintain your blood homocysteine level—this should be between 5 and 9.

• Minimize animal protein, sugar, and saturated fat.

• Increase your intake of dark green leafy vegetables—eat one cup a day of bok choy, escarole, Swiss chard, collard greens, kale, watercress, spinach, or dandelion, mustard, or beet greens.

• Avoid caffeine.

• Limit alcohol to three to five drinks per week.

• Don't smoke.

• Avoid regular use of antacids or acid-blocking medications.

• Eat foods that are high in folic acid, and vitamins $B_6$ and $B_{12}$.

• Take a good vitamin B complex or a good multivitamin.

## Correct Common Nutrient Deficiencies

Vitamins, minerals, and fatty acids all work as a complex team during the millions of biochemical reactions that take place in our bodies every day. The best way to help these processes is to make sure your body has enough of each of the proper nutrients it needs. That's why we take supplements.

Different people at different ages will need more or less of certain nutrients depending on their genetics, health conditions, stress level, environmental exposures, and diet and exercise patterns. A program can be individualized based on an assessment by a qualified health care practitioner or via various blood or urine tests, as well as by symptoms.

In his landmark 1956 book, *Biochemical Individuality,* author Roger Williams showed that our nutritional needs are as unique as our fingerprints. He suggested that some people might need doses of vitamins and minerals far beyond those specified by the RDA. The good news is that most of our needs can be taken care of by a good high-potency multivitamin and mineral supplement.

Below is a brief guide to vitamins and minerals and essential fatty acids.

## Vitamins

Everyone should take a good multivitamin every day. And you must pay attention to whichever vitamins you take. It still surprises us when we read supplement labels and find ingredients such as hydrogenated fats, artificial colorings and flavorings, inert substances, and other unwanted and unnecessary additions. Vitamins and supplements are supposed to be healthful. Why would they contain unhealthful additives?

The truth is that vitamin manufacturers often care more about the bottom line than your health. In order to increase sales, lengthen shelf life, and reduce manufacturing costs, vitamin companies may add unhealthful ingredients to your vitamin tablets, including:

- Artificial sweeteners or flavorings, for improved taste
- Hydrogenated fats, for flavor and longer shelf life

- Artificial colors, for a better appearance
- Glaze, for shine
- Binders, fillers, and flow agents, to make the ingredients flow more smoothly through the tablet-making machinery and make the tablets compress, holding them together longer

What's more, manufacturers often select cheap raw materials that our bodies either can't absorb or can't use, rather than more

---

### ULTRAPREVENTION TIPS FOR HEALTHFUL EATING

- Don't diet! You will slow down your metabolism, lose muscle, obsess about food, and binge after the diet is over.
- Choose high-NCR foods for every meal.
- Whenever possible, eat organic.
- Pay attention to your body's signals of hunger and satiety.
- Develop a rhythm of eating throughout the day, both for meals and snacks.
- If it has a label, either don't eat it, or read the label very carefully to make sure the food inside is good.
- Include a source of high-quality protein at each meal, especially breakfast.
- Don't skip breakfast.
- Include a good source of essential fatty acids daily—fish, flaxseed, and/or nuts.
- Avoid eating three hours or less before bedtime.
- Drink water as your main beverage; aim for 8 to 10 glasses a day.
- Prepare foods in a healthy form—use low-temperature grilling, baking, roasting, steaming, poaching, or sautéing. (Avoid frying or charbroiling.)

---

absorbable and active forms of ingredients. Examples include:
• Synthetic and cheaper vitamin E (called dl-alpha-tocopherol) is used instead of the more expensive but active form of vitamin E (mixed natural tocopherols, or d-alpha-tocopherol).
• Cheaper but less absorbable forms of minerals are added, such as calcium carbonate instead of calcium citrate, calcium citrate-malate, or chelated calcium; or magnesium oxide instead of magnesium glycinate, or chelated magnesium.

Finally, some ingredients in some supplements may be downright dangerous. Recent analyses have shown that many calcium supplements contain excessive amounts of lead. Colloidal minerals obtained from the ocean floor may also contain unwanted amounts of mercury and heavy metals. Some herbal products may contain contaminants or potentially harmful ingredients. A few herbal products have even been found to contain amounts of FDA-controlled prescription medications as unlisted ingredients.

We prefer manufacturers who provide third-party, off-the-shelf assays of their products; these manufacturers are generally more trustworthy than larger corporate manufacturers because by producing smaller lots of supplements, they use fewer unwanted additives (such as flow agents that allow ingredients to pass through high-capacity machines, or preservatives that extend the shelf life). They also tend to make supplements that contain only nutrients, not binders, fillers, flow agents, colorings, flavorings, or preservatives.

For more information on independent assays of commonly available supplements, check with your vitamin manufacturer or go to www.consumerlabs.com.

There are too many vitamins to discuss individually (and we have mentioned many throughout this book), but there are four we want to highlight, because we feel these are necessary but sometimes overlooked.

### 1. Folic acid (a.k.a. folate)

• Take 800 mcg to 1 mg (1,000 mcg) per day.

• Some people may need ten times that amount, depending on their genes. Have your doctor monitor your homocysteine level through a blood test to be sure you're getting adequate amounts.

• Remember that folate from food is not as well absorbed as the folate from supplements, but good sources include black-eyed peas and legumes, leafy dark green vegetables, asparagus, whole grains (rice germ is especially high), nuts—especially walnuts and almonds—and liver.

• Folate is easily destroyed by light or heat, so keep your supplements in a tightly sealed container in a cool place.

### 2. Vitamin $B_6$, or pyridoxine

• Doses in the range of 5 to 10 mg a day of $B_6$ are usually required (the RDA is 2 mg), although some people may need more.

• Be aware that excessive doses (over 500 mg a day) have been linked to peripheral nerve injury or neuropathy.

• Good food sources include sunflower seeds, wheat germ, beans (especially soybeans), walnuts, fish, eggs, and liver.

### 3. Vitamin $B_{12}$ (hydroxycobalamin or methylcobalamin)

• 500 mcg daily is needed for adequate protection from heart disease; however, if you are taking $B_{12}$ orally, much of it is not absorbed and larger doses of up to 1,000 to 2,000 mcg (1 to 2 mg) may be necessary.

• Absorption of $B_{12}$ can be impaired by aging and can occur as a result of digestive disorders and antacid use ($B_{12}$ shots can compensate for those who are having trouble digesting it). Consider increasing your dosage by as much as 50 percent if you are over sixty-five years old.

• Sublingual (under the tongue) forms of $B_{12}$ can also be effective.

• Good food sources include liver, sardines, oily fish, egg yolks, and cheese.

### 4. Trimethylglycine (a.k.a. betaine)

• Betaine is a derivative of amino acids that is essential for proper homocysteine metabolism. It can be supplemented in doses ranging from 500 to 3,000 mg a day.

• There are several good sources of betaine, including legumes, broccoli, spinach, beets, and fish.

## Minerals

Because the body needs many, many minerals, as with vitamins it would take more space than we have here to include the importance of each one. Instead, we will highlight only three: magnesium and zinc, because of their pervasive deficiencies in our diets, and calcium, because it is so critical for our muscle and bone health. It is impossible to be healthy without proper levels of these minerals. Most blood tests are not sensitive enough to detect more subtle deficiencies.

### Magnesium

Magnesium is the relaxation mineral. If you are constipated, have a twitch, a spasm, a cramp, a headache, or an irritation, chances are good you may be low on magnesium, which is critical for over three hundred chemical reactions in the body. Magnesium is also the mineral the average person is most likely to be deficient in.

Magnesium levels are decreased by excess alcohol, salt, coffee, phosphoric acid in colas, profuse sweating, prolonged or intense stress, chronic diarrhea, heavy menstrul flow, and by diuretics (water pills), antibiotics, and other drugs.

Signs and symptoms of conditions associated with magnesium deficiency include irritability, heart flutters or palpitations, frequent headaches, migraines, trouble swallowing, muscle twitching, leg or hand cramps, restless leg syndrome, excess stress, reflux, depression, insomnia, fatigue, constipation, asthma, hypoglycemia, and heart disease. Among the diseases associated with magnesium deficiency are osteoporosis, constipation, congestive heart failure, insulin resistance, diabetes, and kidney stones.

Some of the foods that contain the most magnesium are kelp, wheat bran, millet, dulse, almonds, wheat germ, collard greens, cashews, barley, filberts, pecans, dates, beans, tofu, shrimp, avocado, and soybeans.

More on magnesium:

• The RDA for magnesium is about 300 mg a day. Most of us get far less than 200 mg.

• People with magnesium deficiency will benefit from 400 to 1,000 mg a day. Symptoms, including stress, constipation, insomnia, indigestion, headaches, and muscle twitching, are the best clue to deficiency.

• The most absorbable forms are magnesium glycinate, citrate, taurate, and aspartate. Magnesium malate, succinate, and fumarate are also good.

• Avoid magnesium carbonate, sulfate, gluconate, and oxide. They are less well absorbed (and the cheapest and most common forms found in supplements).

• The most common side effects of oral magnesium supplements are diarrhea, stomach cramps, and gas, which can be reduced if you switch to magnesium glycinate.

• Magnesium is best taken as a team with other minerals in a multimineral formula.

• People with kidney disease or severe heart disease should take magnesium only under a doctor's supervision.

## Zinc

Not only is zinc critical for proper immune function and wound healing, it is also involved in more biochemical bodily reactions than any other mineral. Still, a recent government survey indicated that 73 percent of Americans are deficient in zinc.

The benefits of zinc include healthy immune function; wound healing; maintenance of proper taste, smell, and vision; male sexual function; fertility and prostate health; skin health; and proper digestion (zinc is needed for activation of digestive enzymes). It is also critical in maintaining adequate detoxification and activating a key enzyme needed in every cell to get rid of heavy metals like mercury and lead.

Stress (emotional, physical, or chemical), exposure to heavy metals, pollution, pesticides, and aging can all lead to zinc deficiency. Some of the signs and symptoms or conditions associated with zinc deficiency include: frequent infections, diarrhea, slow wound healing, poor digestion, insulin resistance, impaired taste and poor appetite, impotence, diabetes, skin rashes, enlarged prostate, acne, hair loss, dandruff, bad breath, and eating disorders.

Common food sources of zinc include pecans, Brazil nuts, whole grains, dulse and kelp (seaweed), ginger root, egg yolks, fish, legumes (especially split peas), pumpkin seeds, and oysters (be careful of too many oysters, although they are the best source of zinc, due to contamination from pollutants such as heavy metals, and the risks of contracting hepatitis A).

More on zinc:

- The RDA for zinc is about 15 mg a day.
- The dose for optimal health and therapeutic use can range from 15 mg to 100 mg/day—we recommend 25 to 50 mg a day.
- The total dose should always be kept below 150 mg because of the potential for toxicity.

• Always ensure adequate copper intake during zinc supplementation because zinc and copper compete for absorption in the gut. Excessive zinc supplementation will deplete copper levels, so these minerals should be taken together, usually in a ratio of about 10 to 15 parts zinc to 1 part copper.

• The best forms include zinc sulfate hepahydrate, zinc mono-methionine, and zinc picolinate; zinc aspartate, orotate, and citrate are also effective.

• Take zinc at least two hours before or after eating a lot of fiber; fiber interferes with zinc's absorption.

• Toxic effects from long-term high doses of zinc may include copper deficiency, anemia, low HDL level, and paradoxically low immune function. Acute toxic effects are rare but can include dizziness, vomiting, and lethargy.

• If you are taking it for the treatment of a cold (to shorten its duration), make sure you use zinc gluconate lozenges and take no more than five lozenges during the course of a day.

### Calcium

The body's most abundant mineral is calcium, and over 90 percent of it is stored in our bones. Besides helping to build strong bones, calcium is critical for sound teeth, muscle contraction, nervous system function, heartbeat regulation, blood clotting, and many other critical bodily functions.

We tend to lose calcium through poor diet and health habits, including consuming excess alcohol, caffeine, sugar, phosphoric acid (in colas), salt, excess animal protein, and/or aspartame. Reduced stomach acid from antacids or acid-blocking drugs (Prilosec, Prevacid, Aciphex, Nexium, Protonix) prevents adequate calcium absorption as well.

Unfortunately, we have been brainwashed to believe that the best (and only) source of calcium is milk or dairy products. As noted earlier, there are several problems with milk; regardless, calcium from other sources is actually better absorbed.

Other food sources of calcium include seaweed such as kelp (which contains a whopping 1,093 mg of calcium per 100 grams), mustard greens, turnip greens, bok choy, bean sprouts, collard greens, spinach, canned sardines with bones, canned mackerel with bones, sesame seeds, almonds, chestnuts, filberts, walnuts, tofu, soybeans, and garbanzo beans.

More on calcium:

• The RDA for calcium is between 800 and 1,200 mg, an amount that is achievable through diet if you add some of the above calcium-rich sources.

• If you take a calcium supplement, look for calcium citrate-malate, or calcium citrate—but not calcium carbonate, which is the mostly commonly marketed form. Calcium carbonate is a powerful antacid, and remember that acid is needed for proper absorption of minerals. Excess calcium carbonate has been associated with kidney stones.

• Make sure your calcium is in a form that is not too tightly packed. As an experiment, soak a tablet in six ounces of vinegar for half an hour. It should begin to dissolve.

• Calcium can cause constipation. If you are experiencing constipation, try to get more calcium from foods and less from pills. Also, be sure to add magnesium along with calcium to your supplement program.

• Signs of calcium deficiency include weak muscles, high blood pressure, and osteoporosis.

### Essential Fatty Acids

The best way to eat most of your fat is in the form of extra virgin olive oil, fish, flax, nuts, and seeds, with minimal amounts of properly processed (expeller-pressed) vegetable oils. Include only small amounts of saturated fat from animal foods. Stay away from trans fats entirely.

To eat foods high in essential fatty acids, choose:

- Wild fish: The best sources are small cold-water fish that don't contain high levels of heavy metals and other contaminants. Healthy fish choices include sardines, herring, mackerel, salmon, trout, and arctic char.
- Wild game: Wild elk and deer, and other wild game, are rich sources of omega-3 fats because of the wild plants that they eat.
- Nuts: Walnuts, hazelnuts, pecans, almonds, Brazil nuts, and most others (except for peanuts) contain small amounts of beneficial omega-3 fats. They are also good sources of monounsaturated fats.
- Flaxseed: The seed of flax contains the highest levels of essential fats in the plant kingdom. The flaxseeds must be ground in order for you to digest and absorb the essential oils in them. Organic, pre-ground flaxseed can be bought in most health food stores. The whole seeds can also be ground in a coffee grinder half a cup at a time and stored in a tightly sealed glass container in the fridge. Use on salads, soups, grains, or other foods. Try to eat one to two tablespoons a day.
- Evening primrose, borage, and blackcurrant seed oil: These can be bought as liquid oils or capsules and have high levels of GLA (gamma-linolenic acid), which complements the benefits of omega-3 fats. Though not technically essential fatty acids, these are the good omega-6 fats.

## 2. REPAIR AND ENHANCE DETOXIFICATION

All of us could use a tune-up for our waste and toxin elimination systems. The key systems of elimination are our digestive tract, liver, kidneys, and skin. In order to enhance detoxification, we need to boost the detoxification capacity of each of these organs.

### Digestive tract

Increasing fiber intake and increasing normal bowel frequency enhances elimination of unwanted toxins from our bodies. High-fiber intake has also been associated with lower cholesterol, as well as lower rates of obesity, diabetes, and colon cancer.

### Liver

Specific foods and nutrients in supplement form can support the liver's detoxification process and enhance the elimination of harmful and carcinogenic compounds.

### Kidneys

Because humans are predominantly composed of water (about 66 percent by weight for men, about 60 percent for women), maintaining a continuous intake of clean water and a high rate of urine flow from the kidneys enhances the elimination of unwanted water-soluble compounds.

### Skin

The skin is the largest organ of our bodies by weight. Besides protecting us from the outside world and helping to maintain a constant internal temperature and environment, our skin is an active organ of detoxification. Not only does the skin eliminate wastes through the process of sweating, but it completely regenerates itself once a month. The outer layers of skin are constantly being shed, while new layers are being formed below. This shedding process also results in elimination of unwanted compounds from the body.

Here's how to repair and enhance detoxification:

### 1. Increase your intake of fiber

Increase slowly and aim for 25 to 50 grams of fiber daily (see page 271 for good sources). Use these stool guidelines to adjust your fiber intake for the desired results:

## FAT TIPS

- Reduce the total amount of fat in your diet to 20 to 30 percent (or about 400 to 600 calories, based on 2,000 calories per day).
- No more than 5 percent of the fat you consume should be saturated.
- Eliminate trans fats or partially hydrogenated fat from your diet.
- Avoid refined vegetable oils.
- Have a serving or two of foods containing essential fats daily.
- Add one tablespoon of organic flaxseed and borage oil daily to food, or try 1 to 2 tablespoons of organic ground flaxseed on your food.
- Try three months of a fish oil supplement with DHA and EPA (about 1,000 mg a day) to see how it affects your health for the better, including your skin, hair, and nails.
- If you are taking supplemental fatty acids, make sure you are also taking at least 400 to 800 IU of vitamin E to prevent oxidation of the fats in your system. Essential fats are susceptible to oxidation, and supplements should be kept refrigerated in a tightly sealed, airtight container.
- Make sure you take a high-potency multivitamin and mineral supplement that contains all the nutrients for essential fatty acid metabolism, including vitamin C, vitamin $B_6$, vitamin $B_3$, zinc, and magnesium.
- Choose only high-quality oils, and make sure they are certified organic and are expeller pressed (a process that doesn't damage the oils extracted from vegetable sources). Avoid oils that do not state the method of extraction, or have a bitter aftertaste or rancid flavor.

• Frequency: at least one and up to three formed movements a day (fewer than one a day is considered constipation and increases your risk for cancer and even Parkinson's disease).
• Texture: bulky, soft, and easy to pass
• Tendency to float (indicating a high-fiber content).
• Medium to light brown in color.

## 2. Increase your intake of clean, filtered water
Water intake needs to be *at least* 64 ounces per day. This bare minimum intake represents the amount of water lost by an average-sized person in a single day. Increase your intake of water above this amount to meet the following guidelines:

• Normal urine output should be two to three liters a day (admittedly, few of us actually measure).
• Urine should be mostly clear or with only a slight tinge of yellow (although for those taking vitamins, riboflavin—vitamin $B_2$—causes bright yellow urine).
• Urine should have only a slight to mild odor (unless you eat asparagus, which can impart a pungent odor in people who have a common variation in liver detoxification enzymes).

## 3. Sweat on a regular basis
We recommend aerobic exercise for at least thirty minutes four days per week to a level that causes sweating. In addition to exercise, boost your skin's detoxification capability by using a steam bath or sauna an additional two or three times weekly.

## 4. Increase your intake of foods that boost the liver's detoxification capabilities
These foods provide the liver with the nutrients it needs to process and detoxify unwanted chemicals.

• Eat at least one cup of cruciferous vegetables daily (broccoli, cauliflower, brussels sprouts, cabbage, kale, bok choy).

• Include as much garlic as possible in your diet—or take it as a supplement.

• Eat high-quality sulfur-containing proteins: eggs, whey protein (obtainable in health food stores), garlic, and onions.

• Drink decaffeinated green tea in the morning.

• Try fresh vegetable juices, including carrot, celery, beet, parsley, and ginger.

• Season food with rosemary, which contains carnosol, a potent booster of detoxification enzymes.

• Eat grapes, berries, and citrus fruits, which contain helpful bioflavonoids.

• Try dandelion greens, which help liver detoxification, improve the flow of bile, and increase urine flow.

• Add cilantro to meals; it can help remove heavy metals. Add dark green leafy vegetables, which contain chlorophyll, a helpful detoxifier.

• Get curcuminoids from spices such as turmeric.

• Try herbal detoxification teas containing mixtures of burdock root, dandelion root, ginger root, licorice root, sarsaparilla root, cardamom seed, cinnamon bark, and other herbs.

## 3. Repair the Rust: Oil the Oxidative Stress System

### Antioxidant Foods

Among the many classifications of food is a new one—ORAC, or oxygen radical absorbence capacity, a measurement of the ability of a food to mop up free radicals.

To measure ORAC, scientists put a person's blood in a test tube, add some toxins, and measure how well it takes care of the damage—the higher the ORAC score, the better. (Your doctor is not likely to test for ORAC, but specialty labs will do it.)

The best way to increase your blood ORAC is to eat eight to ten servings of high-NCR vegetables and fruits a day. The superstars in the ORAC world are:

- Berries such as blueberries and blackberries
- Garlic
- Kale
- Spinach
- Brussels sprouts
- Plums
- Broccoli florets
- Beets
- Oranges
- Tomatoes

Notice that antioxidant-rich foods are also frequently brightly colored. Some of these pigment antioxidants include:

- Carotenes, such as beta-, alpha-, and gamma-carotene
- Lycopene (present in red foods, such as tomatoes)
- Other carotenoids, such as lutein, astaxanthin, and zeaxanthin
- Polyphenols (in green tea)
- Anthocyanidins (in berries, beets, and grapes)
- Quercetin (found in fruit and vegetable rinds)
- Curcuminoids (such as in turmeric)
- Trans-resveratrol (from grapes and red wine, especially cabernet)

### Take Antioxidant Minerals and Vitamins

We've already discussed multivitamins, but another issue of concern with supplements is making sure they contain the right antioxidants. The big players here include vitamin A, the carotenoids (beta- and alpha-carotene, lutein, lycopene, and xeanthin), the tocopherols (the vitamin E family), vitamin C, vitamin D, the B-complex vitamins, zinc, and selenium. A good vitamin that takes care of your anti-oxidant issues will offer:

• Vitamin A: 5,000 to 10,000 IU/day. Vitamin A is also known as retinol and comes from animal sources such as fish oils, liver, eggs, and fortified dairy products. It is a great free radical fighter, but do not take too much without a doctor's supervision—high amounts can cause liver damage, bone loss, and birth defects. The RDA for pregnant women is 2,700 IU. Pregnant women should take no more than 8,000 IU a day from all sources. If you prefer, you can get your vitamin A through mixed carotenoids (15,000 to 25,000 IU/day). Carotenoids are found in vegetables, and our bodies can convert them into vitamin A. There are many different kinds of carotenoids found in yellow and orange fruits and vegetables. Many of these can now be found as a blend in supplements, including beta- and alpha-carotene, lutein, lycopene, and xeanthin.

• Mixed tocopherols (vitamin E): 400 to 800 IU/day. Vitamin E is found in many forms, including d-alpha, gamma, and delta.

---

### LYMPHATIC FLOW AND DETOXIFICATION

Our lymphatic system (which includes the lymph nodes as well as the small ducts connecting them) is the path through which our bodies recirculate fluids from our tissues back to the heart and kidneys. Healthy lymphatic flow speeds the elimination of toxins from our bodies. To improve the flow:

• Exercise (especially swimming).
• Get a massage.
• Bounce on a rebounder or mini-trampoline. The action can have profound effects on lymph flow and circulation.
• Take regular saunas or steam baths.

---

• Vitamin C: 250 to 2,000 mg/day. One the most important and well-known antioxidants.

• Vitamin D: 400 to 1,200 IU/day.

• Vitamin B complex: a blend of the eight B vitamins, including thiamine ($B_1$), 25 to 100 mg; riboflavin ($B_2$), 25 to 100 mg; niacin ($B_3$), 25 to 100 mg; pyridoxine ($B_6$), 15 to 100 mg; folic acid ($B_9$), 800 mcg; cyanocobalamin ($B_{12}$), 500 to 1,000 mcg; pantothenic acid ($B_5$), 100 to 500 mg; and biotin, 500 to 1,000 mg.

• Zinc: 25 to 50 mg/day. As mentioned above, take copper with your zinc at a ratio of 15:1 zinc to copper.

• Selenium: 100 to 200 mcg/day. This dose works to help recycle our major antioxidant, glutathione.

## Consume Herbal and Phytochemical Antioxidants

These are best taken as a regular part of our diet, but sometimes can be added as supplements when extra antioxidant protection is indicated. Some have specific benefits for different systems in the body, such as hawthorn (for the heart), ginkgo (for the brain), or milk thistle (for the liver).

Follow the guidance of an experienced practitioner unless otherwise indicated here for specific problems. Herbal antioxidants include:

• Ashwaganda—(*Withania somnifera*), an ancient Ayurvedic or Indian ginsenglike herb.

• Chocolate (*Theobroma cacao*)—unfortunately, this must be taken in large doses to be effective and is usually found with sugar and dairy products added.

• Cranberry (*Vaccinium macrocarpon*)

• Garlic (*Allium sativum*)

• Ginkgo (*Ginkgo biloba*)

• Ginger (*Zingiber officinale*)

• Green tea (*Camellia sinensis*)

- Grape seed (*Vitus vinifera*)
- Hawthorn (*Crataegus oxycantha*)
- Horse chestnut (*Aesculus hippocastanum*)
- Milk thistle (*Silybum marianum*)
- Purple grape (*Vitis labrusca*)
- Rosemary (*Rosmarinus officinalis*)
- Turmeric (*Curcuma longa*)

## Other Rust-Fighting Therapies

### Exercise

Regular aerobic exercise is a powerful way to boost the body's rust-fighting capacity. When you exercise on a regular basis, your body makes more of the powerful rust-fighting antioxidants such as catalase, superoxide dismutase (SOD), and glutathione peroxidase. These natural antioxidants are some of the most important and powerful substances made by our bodies. They are normally created to sop up free radicals released during the process of energy (ATP) production.

However, too much exercise, or worse, the weekend warrior syndrome (alternating between channel surfing during the week and sporadic, intense exercise on the weekend), can actually increase oxidative stress. Most of us, of course, won't get too much exercise—that's only likely to occur in professional or competitive athletes. The infrequent exerciser's body has not been primed for vigorous workouts because of a lack of regular exercise. When the weekend warrior then engages in vigorous exercise, free radical production again outstrips antioxidant capacity.

### Hydration

Dehydration can cause all types of symptoms, including dry skin, fatigue, headaches, dizziness, painful and stiff joints, constipation, and even frequent infections. The hydration state of our cells is closely related to our nutrient status, hormone balance, and oxidative stress levels. Changes in our water level can affect cellular metabolism, and all the biochemical signals needed for optimal health. So remember to drink to your health and drink heavily and heartily—water, that is: at least eight glasses of pure, clean water every day.

## Sleep

Sleep deprivation has been shown to reduce levels of glutathione (our major antioxidant) in the hormonal command center of the brain. The optimal dose of sleep has not yet been fully established; different people require different amounts.

The best way to keep your circadian, or daily, rhythms in balance is to keep regular sleeping and waking habits (as well as regular eating, exercising, and resting habits). Living a chaotic lifestyle with erratic patterns in any of the above can lead to many problems, only one of which is increased oxidative stress, which, in turn, leads to poor sleep.

## Detoxification and Inflammation

Two of the most important causes of oxidative stress are an overwhelmed detoxification system and out-of-control inflammation. Addressing these two forces of illness with our ultraprevention program will also reduce the amount of oxidative stress. Please follow our guidelines for waste and heat.

## 4. REPAIR IMMUNE FUNCTION AND REDUCE INFLAMMATION

## Eat Anti-inflammatory Foods

Food, our eating habits, and our weight play an important role in determining the degree of inflammation in our bodies. Certain foods can trigger and magnify inflammation, while others reduce and reverse it. Gaining weight tends to create inflammation, while losing weight tends to reduce it.

The entire ultraprevention approach to food, nutrition, and eating is designed to reduce inflammation and oxidative stress. In order to maximize the rewards of the ultraprevention program, for these two weeks you should increase your intake of anti-inflammatory foods, while decreasing your intake of inflammatory foods.

Here are some specific guidelines:

A. Follow the nutritional guidelines outlined above in the "Repair" section starting on page 268.
B. Follow the instructions for the elimination diet in the "Repair the Digestive System" section on page 269.
C. Add the following anti-inflammatory foods (most of which you should already be eating):

- Starches: nongluten grains, including brown rice, millet, quinoa, amaranth, teff, tapioca, and buckwheat
- Fruits: unsweetened fresh fruit
- Fish and meat: fresh fish, including salmon, halibut, cod, sole, trout; wild game; lean chicken and beef
- Legumes: peas, beans, and lentils
- Nuts and seeds: almonds, cashews, walnuts, pecans, hazelnuts, Brazil nuts, sesame seeds (tahini), sunflower and pumpkin seeds, and nut butters made of these
- Dairy products: Drink only milk alternatives, such as soy, rice, or almond milk. Or drink low- or nonfat varieties; the same is true for solid dairy products such as yogurt.
- Vegetables: Eat almost everything! Eat them raw, or steam, sauté, juice, or bake them.
- Fats: olive oil, flaxseed oil, and expeller-pressed sunflower, sesame, walnut, pumpkin, or almond oil

- Beverages: Drink at least eight glasses of filtered or distilled water a day; herbal teas are also good
- Spices and herbs: cinnamon, cumin, turmeric, garlic, ginger, dill, oregano, parsley, rosemary, coriander, tarragon, and thyme
- Sweeteners: keep them to a minimum, but you can use fruit sweeteners or brown rice syrup

## Avoid the following inflammatory foods:

- Starches: any form of wheat, oats, spelt, rye, kamut, barley, and products containing gluten
- Seafood: shellfish, including shrimp, lobster, crayfish, clams, oysters, mussels, and scallops
- Meat: beef, pork, cold cuts, frankfurters, sausage, canned meats
- Nuts: pistachios, peanuts, and peanut butter
- Dairy products: milk, cheese, cottage cheese, yogurt, cream, butter, ice cream, frozen yogurt, nondairy creamers
- Fats: margarine, shortening, trans fats, processed oils, butter, commercial salad dressings and spreads
- Beverages: alcohol, coffee, black tea, sodas, and any caffeinated drinks
- Sweeteners: brown and white sugar, honey, maple syrup, corn syrup, and high-fructose corn syrup

### Include special anti-inflammatory nutrients
The plant world has graced us with all manner of healing compounds. Use these freely in cooking and you will do much toward keeping inflammation in check.

Here are additional natural anti-inflammatory nutrients and where they can be found:

- Bromelain (found in pineapple)
- Capsaicin (cayenne)

- Carnosol and carnosic acid (rosemary)
- Carvacrol (oregano)
- Curcumin (turmeric)
- Gingerol, shagaol (ginger)
- Trans-resveratrol (purple grapes)
- Thymol (thyme)
- Quercetin (onions, apples, tea)

## Additional Measures: Improving Your Lifestyle

Lifestyle factors play an enormous role in mediating inflammation and immune function. Dr. Candice Pert, of the National Institutes of Health, has discovered that our immune cells receive chemical messages directly from our brains. These are the "molecules of emotion" chronicled in Dr. Pert's 1997 book of the same name. Next time you have a feeling or thought, remember that your immune system is listening.

Feelings have the power to heal and the power to harm. For example, researchers have found that medical students' immune cell function prior to taking exams became impaired (as measured by the activity of immune system cells known as lymphocytes and natural killer cells). An even more dramatic negative effect appeared in those most worried about their performance.

On the other hand, the mind can perform miracles of healing. In fact, the chemicals produced during deep relaxation, as well as moments of joy and laughter, are powerful anticancer and infection-fighting compounds that drug companies spend millions of dollars trying to imitate. Thus you have access every moment of the day to the world's greatest pharmacy—your mind.

Laughter is also potent medicine. At Loma Linda University, researchers examined more than ten different markers of immune function, including natural killer cells (cells that are the security police of your immune system, searching out and killing cancer cells and virally infected cells), lymphocyte activity, and cytokines.

They drew blood from a group of medical students, and had them watch a funny video for one hour. They again drew blood, thirty and ninety minutes later, and then twelve hours after, and discovered that thanks to the video, the students' immune systems were boosted.

Many mind-body techniques can be used to reduce inflammation and balance and strengthen your immune system. Find something that works for you and practice it daily, even if only for fifteen minutes. Here are some of the best measures (some of which we discussed in Step Three):

- Meditation
- Yoga
- Breathing techniques
- Guided imagery
- Journaling
- Psychotherapy
- Prayer
- Hypnosis
- Support groups
- Laughter

### Exercise and Inflammation

While excessive or sudden strenuous exercise can cause acute inflammation, a regular and consistent exercise program is a potent tool for reducing inflammation. This may explain why long-term regular exercise dramatically reduces heart disease, a condition we now know to be a disease of inflammation.

A dramatic study described in the *Journal of American Medicine* (May 12, 1999) showed that after six months of exercising, volunteers had lower levels of a broad range of inflammatory molecules in their systems and an increase in anti-inflammatory molecules.

In another recent study of almost six thousand men and women, researchers examined the relationship between physical activity and markers of inflammation in a healthy elderly population; they found that exercisers all had lower levels of the markers of inflammation.

Many other studies have found a positive connection between exercise, inflammation, and aging. These reveal that exercise reduces the markers of inflammation, indicating a generalized anti-inflammatory effect.

## Massage

Touch is healing. We intuitively recognize the power of touch to heal when we stroke our ailing children's foreheads, or rub a part of our body that is sore. Now we have science to back up ancient practices.

For example, in neonatal care units across the country, TAC-TIC therapy (touching and caressing, tender in caring) is gaining a foothold because of its profound effects on weight gain, immune function, and cardiovascular health in infants.

HIV-positive patients who received daily massages for one month showed a significant increase in the number of their natural killer cells, and some white blood cells, as well as a significant decrease in cortisol (the stress hormone). And in ulcer patients, deep massage was found to be equal in relief to their routine medications.

Regular touching and massage can increase communication between the brain and the immune system, reducing overall inflammation. Although science does not yet fully comprehend the reasons, these effects may be related to increased blood and lymph circulation, as well as the simple act of being touched.

## Weight Loss: Insulin Resistance and Inflammation

We all know that there are not too many three-hundred-pound eighty-five-year-olds walking around. Simply being overweight itself causes inflammation. The fat cells seem to produce an inflammatory cytokine called IL-6, or interleukin 6, and overweight people (particularly those apple-shaped, with fat around the middle) seem to have higher levels of C-reactive protein. Inflammation is routinely found in diabetics, and sugar itself seems to trigger inflammation. The process by which this occurs is being unraveled. Correcting imbalances in blood sugar and insulin plays a critical role in controlling inflammation as we age.

## 5. REPAIR METABOLISM

### Repair Your Mitochondria

During the first two weeks of the ultraprevention plan (the "Remove" phase), you learned to remove obstacles to perfect your metabolism. Now, during the "Repair" phase, we are repairing your mitochondria, balancing your blood sugar and your hormones, and boosting your thyroid function.

The most effective way to increase the size, efficiency, and number of mitochondria is through regular exercise. (For more on the importance of mitochondria, see page 193).

One of the best ways to measure mitochondrial function is a test called the cardiometabolic stress test, which, unfortunately, few doctors can provide. At Canyon Ranch, however, we use it often; we put patients on a treadmill and strap a mask on them that measures how much oxygen they consume and how much carbon dioxide they release while working out. The more oxygen you can consume or breathe per minute, the better your mitochondria are working.

As you remember, we are measuring VO2 max, or the maximum amount of oxygen used per minute. This number is actually a very good predictor of mortality. If you have a low VO2 max, which indicates lazy mitochondria, your risk of premature death is higher than average (refer back to page 197 for more on VO2 max).

Our exercise recommendations:

• Perform aerobic exercise for thirty minutes four days a week. To qualify as aerobic, you must either break a sweat, or reach and/or stay within your target heart range for at least twenty minutes. Your target heart range is between 70 and 85 percent of your maximum heart rate (calculated as 220 minus your age).

• Include interval training (high-intensity bursts of exercise) in your aerobic workout at least three times weekly. This can significantly boost your metabolism.

• Do resistance (strength) training two to three days per week for twenty minutes. You should feel at least a bit sore the following day. Resistance training means pushing or pulling against resistance, or lifting your own weight against gravity. This usually requires the use of weights, Dynabands, or other equipment to provide resistance.

## Balance Your Blood Sugar

• Eat every three to four hours (three meals, two snacks). Smaller amounts eaten more frequently keep your blood sugar and insulin levels normal. Two things raise your blood sugar—foods that quickly turn to sugar when you eat them, and large quantities of any food.

• Eliminate the White Menace. Avoid low-NCR carbohydrates.

• Increase fiber (slowly) to 30 to 50 grams per day. Use predominantly soluble fiber, such as broccoli and greens, or beans—try bean dip, hummus, beans in salads and soups.

• Reduce or eliminate starchy root vegetables (potatoes, turnips, parsnips) and amylose-containing grains (wheat, rye, barley, oats, rice)—amylose is a starch that can block the body's metabolic thermostat.

• Include protein and good fat with every meal or snack. Breakfast is especially important—start every day with some protein as it helps regulate blood sugar and reduces hunger. Eggs and yogurt can be good choices.

• Eat omega-3 fats regularly—at least one to three servings of fish weekly.

• Eat one to two tablespoons of ground flaxseed daily.

• Reduce saturated fat from animal foods (meat, poultry, dairy fat).

• Strictly eliminate hydrogenated fat (margarine, shortening, all processed and refined oils, and any fried foods).

• Avoid eating three hours or less before bed.

• Eliminate alcohol, or limit it to no more than 3 to 5 glasses of red wine a week.

• Eat no artificial sweeteners or junk food—artificial sweeteners can trigger insulin response from brain signals and fuel sweet cravings.

• Avoid caffeine—it increases the stress hormones and adrenaline, which causes a spike in blood sugar.

• Follow the guidelines for managing stress in the next section. Persistent, unrelieved stress commonly aggravates blood sugar and insulin levels.

• Follow the exercise guidelines above in "Repair Your Mitochondria."

• Take a high-potency multivitamin and mineral supplement.

### Boost Your Thyroid Function

The thyroid produces two different, crucial hormones, known as T4 (thyroxin) and T3 (triiodothyronine). The two basic differences between these are:

• T4 has four iodine molecules attached, while T3 has only three.

• T3 is the more potent, active form of the hormone. It is created from T4 when our bodies remove one of its iodine molecules. This conversion process takes place both in the thyroid gland itself, and in many of our tissues and organs, particularly the liver.

For proper thyroid hormone formation and function, the thyroid requires raw materials to make T3 and T4, as well as the ability to create them. These materials are:

• Tyrosine, a basic amino acid
• Iodine, the key mineral used in producing thyroid hormones. Iodine is found in all seafood and sea vegetables, as well as in iodized salt.
• Selenium, needed to make the active hormone T3 from T4. We recommend 100 to 200 mcg/day from all sources.
• Rosemary (carnosic acid)

Additional factors that impair T4 to T3 conversion are:

• Stress
• The adrenal hormone cortisol
• Fasting and dieting
• Environmental toxins, including petrochemicals such as pesticides and heavy metals such as mercury

# STEP THREE: RECHARGE—THE THIRD TWO WEEKS

**GOALS:**
1. RESTORE NORMAL SLEEP
2. MOVE YOUR BODY
3. PRACTICE STRESS MANAGEMENT
4. PRACTICE OTHER ULTRAPREVENTION TECHNIQUES

The restoration of vitality isn't just about the right diet and supplements. We must also care for the more subtle aspects of our being. How we do this varies from person to person, but each one of us must find the right rhythm for our lives to help us heal properly.

After years of denying the importance of nontangible, nonphysical aspects of healing, science has come around to seeing advantages in such practices as prayer, meditation, movement, touch, and proper breathing. These aspects of healing form the basis for the last part of our ultraprevention program.

Your cells and your genes respond on a moment-to-moment basis not just to your diet and your environment, but to each thought and feeling, each belief, each action taken that supports or depletes your life energy. Medical literature is replete with descriptions of phenomena that defy medical explanation, from spontaneous remissions to successful long-distance prayer. Research has also provided explanation for, and proven the benefits of, practices Western medicine has long considered ineffective, from acupuncture to osteopathy.

But we feel there is more than this mind-body connection that is being debated in science. We believe there is something called a *mindbody*, one whole organism, intimately integrated and coordinated, that cannot be separated into parts.

The boundaries we have created by saying that the mind somehow influences the body, or that the body influences the mind, distort our perception of how our bodies and minds actually function. Trying to divide mind and body is like trying to divide yin and yang. Neither can stand alone; together they make one totality.

The complex links between our brain chemistry, immune system, and hormones regulate and direct almost all the actions of our bodies. Those rhythms are intricately linked to how we live our lives, how we sleep, and the ways in which we move our bodies, nourish our souls, and create our environments, as well as the sounds we hear and the images we see.

Over the past few years the number of texts on all of these subjects has burgeoned. We cannot pretend that we can cover this subject completely here. What we will provide is a brief overview of the components of healing that involve these more subtle aspects of health, as well as specific guidelines for practices that can restore your health and create a vibrant environment in which your cells, and your soul, can flourish.

We are not encouraging you to change your belief systems or suggesting that all of the following practices are exactly right for you. We are suggesting that, for two weeks, you open your mind and try out some specific behaviors that have been scientifically proven to alter your biochemistry and physiology and that can create happy brain chemicals, as well as healing hormones and anti-inflammatory molecules.

Creating a rhythm to your life and your day, moving your body, exploring your breath, surrounding yourself with certain wavelengths of light and frequencies of sound, being touched and massaged—all these can profoundly influence your health. Their power often exceeds that of any change in diet or supplements.

A coordinated effort to integrate these practices—slowly at first, and then more fully as you grow comfortable—will lead you to the buoyant and zestful life you deserve.

## 1. RESTORE NORMAL SLEEP

Research suggests that 70 percent of Americans are sleep-deprived. The era of coffee bars has been joined by the era of prescription stimulants to keep people awake and functioning. We live in a world where multitasking is now the norm, where doing five things at once is considered not just desirable but often necessary.

Is this really a good thing? No. Our bodies' biological rhythms evolved along with the rhythms of day and night, which are used to signal a whole cascade of hormonal and neurochemical reactions that repair our DNA, build tissues and muscle, and regulate weight and mood chemicals. The advent of the lightbulb changed all that. Now we lead 24/7 lives and consider ourselves lucky if we manage to get seven hours of restful sleep a night.

But when our rhythms are disturbed by inadequate or insufficient sleep, disease and breakdown gain the upper hand. Most of all, our adrenal glands pump out extra amounts of cortisol, with all its harmful effects, including brain damage and dementia, weight gain, diabetes, heart attacks, high blood pressure, depression, osteoporosis, depressed immunity, and more.

By adhering to the following guidelines, you can help restore your natural sleep rhythm. It may take more than two weeks, but using these tools in a coordinated way will eventually reset your biological rhythms.

### Create an aesthetic environment

Decorate your bedroom with serene and restful colors (shades of blue, pink, pale oatmeal, or deep purple seem to create serenity and calm), and eliminate clutter and distractions. Relaxing surroundings can help your mind relax, too.

## Consider a sleep ritual

Sleep isn't something you should do between eating, socializing, and watching TV. In order to sleep well, you must work a little at it. Create a special set of small tasks (such as saying a prayer, writing in a journal, or performing a relaxation exercise) that you can do to help ready your system physically and psychologically for bed. This can guide your body into a deep, healing sleep.

## Practice regular rhythms of sleep

Go to bed and wake up at the same time each day. At first this may be difficult, but eventually you can and will awake without an alarm clock.

## Use your bed for sleep and sex only

This means no reading or watching television. Using your bed for eating, working, watching television, or sending e-mail from your laptop creates a conditioned response of wakefulness. Much like Pavlov's dogs, your sleep rhythm can be conditioned by external cues; keeping your bed for sleeping goes a long way toward setting up the right signals.

## If you wake up, walk away

Leave your bed if you awaken in the middle of the night and can't easily get back to sleep. Return only when you are ready. Do not force yourself to sleep. The more you try, the more you will stimulate your brain, and you will have an even harder time falling asleep.

## Keep your room dust-free

Many people are allergic to dust, which can create nasal congestion and lead to trouble breathing. If you wake feeling stuffed up, consider getting a HEPA or ULPA air filter for your bedroom.

### Create total darkness

Your brain's pineal gland is its control center for melatonin, which regulates sleep and wakefulness. It wants complete darkness at night. So remember that your eyelids are only opaque, not lightproof. Remove an obtrusive luminescent clock from your bedroom; even a night-light can be stimulating and disturb the hormonal rhythms necessary for healing and repair and healthy aging. Consider special white-out shades and window covers, or eye shades.

### Rid yourself of distracting noise

White-noise machines can be effective in keeping away unwanted noises. Earplugs are another great invention that can reduce unavoidable sounds at night. Though we may not be conscious of noise, our brain registers it, and it may prevent us from deep and healing sleep.

### Avoid caffeine

While coffee seems to keep us awake and ward off sleepiness, recent research suggests that, paradoxically, it leads to an increase in daytime sleepiness, leading to increased caffeine consumption and a dangerous spiral of disturbed biological rhythms that include difficulty falling asleep, reduced sleep efficiency, and significant metabolic and mood effects, including depression.

### Avoid alcohol

Although it initially acts as a depressant and may help you fall asleep, alcohol can cause you to wake within a few hours. It also affects the quality of your sleep, which will be disturbed, contributing to a hangover. Alcohol can worsen other conditions, including sleep apnea and restless leg syndrome (nighttime muscle twitching). Alcohol also interferes with normal sleep patterns and can decrease REM sleep, leading to a chaotic rhythm and all its attendant ills. If you are having trouble sleeping, or are tired in the day, try avoiding alcohol altogether for a few months and see what happens.

### Get regular exposure to daylight

Do this for at least twenty minutes a day. Sunlight triggers the brain to release specific chemicals and hormones, such as melatonin, that are vital to healthy sleep, mood, and aging. In one study, melatonin levels of institutionalized people who had no exposure to natural light were higher in the day than at night (the reverse of what they should be), and such elevated levels indicated an increase in sleep and mood disorders. The bright sun tells our brain to shut off the melatonin during the day. Without it, our brains can malfunction, leading to sleeping disturbances as well as changes in appetite and mood, aging, and even the promotion and growth of cancer cells.

### Eat no later than three hours before bed

Eating a heavy meal prior to bed can lead to a bad night's sleep. Even if you do sleep, you are more likely to get reflux, nightmares, and feel sluggish in the morning.

### Avoid physical activity late in the evening

Exercise should be completed at least two hours before going to bed (any time before that is fine, morning, afternoon, or early evening). Though exercise earlier in the day can reduce insomnia and improve sleep quality, exercising right before bed will increase endorphins and other mood- and energy-boosting chemicals that can make it difficult to fall asleep.

### Take hot salt and soda aromatherapy baths

A hot bath relaxes muscles and reduces tension. Adding a half to one cup of Epsom salts (magnesium sulfate) and the same amount of baking soda (sodium bicarbonate) to your bath will give you the benefits of magnesium absorbed through your skin, and the alkaline-balancing effects of the baking soda, both of which aid sleep. Aromatherapy, too, can induce relaxation hormones in the brain and reduce cortisol levels. Add ten drops of a soothing essential oil such as lavender, vanilla, or sandalwood to your bath.

### Get a massage before bed
Or perform self-massage or do a short stretching routine. These techniques help reduce tension in the body, and increase circulation and the triggering of the relaxation response.

### Use a heating pad on your solar plexus
Warming yourself just beneath the navel raises your core temperature. This helps trigger the proper chemistry for sleep. A hot water bottle, a heating pad, or another person's warm body can do the trick.

### If possible, avoid medications that interfere with sleep
Sedatives treat insomnia well on a short-term basis, but they can ultimately lead to dependence and disruption of normal sleep rhythms.

### Play a relaxation tape or CD
Relaxation exercises, including guided imagery, progressive muscle relaxation, or autogenic training, can help calm the mind and relax the body, inducing a deep and restful sleep.

### Take relaxing minerals
Taking 300 to 500 mg of magnesium and calcium before bed can help you relax and provide you with a deeper and more restful sleep.

### Try herbal therapies

Many herbs have been studied in the treatment of sleep disorders. Try valerian root extract (as directed on the bottle) one hour before bed. Other helpful herbs include kava kava, passionflower, and lemon balm. Experiment with herbal combinations or blends to find the best effect for you.

### Consider testing

The most common sleep disorder (and most underdiagnosed) is sleep apnea. If you experience excessive daytime sleepiness, fatigue, snoring, and have been seen to stop breathing in the middle of the night by a partner, you could be one of the many undiagnosed sufferers of this condition. Your risk of increased blood pressure and heart disease is high; diagnosis and treatment are necessary. Get an overnight sleep study done in a sleep lab. It might just save your life!

## 2. MOVE YOUR BODY

As a race, humans have never been more sedentary in our history, and never before have we had so many epidemics related to lack of movement, from obesity to diabetes, from heart disease to depression.

The benefits of exercise are too numerous to mention—many of them have already been discussed vis à vis a reduction in inflammation and oxidative stress, improvement in detoxification, and normalization of hormonal and metabolic rhythms. If there were a magic pill that could prevent most of the ills of our civilization, it might be exercise—in fact, it is one of the best antidotes to the five forces of illness.

If you want proof, exercise regularly. You will see and feel the results. For example, a recent study of men older than fifty found that with appropriate training they could achieve the same fitness level as twenty-year-olds. A Finnish study (*New England Journal of*

*Medicine,* April 9, 1998) of more than seven thousand men and women found that those who didn't exercise much were four times as likely to die as those who did. And in his landmark study of two decades ago on aging and exercise, Stanford's Dr. James Fries found that "not only do persons with better health habits [exercise, maintaining a healthy weight, and avoiding smoking] survive longer, but in such persons, disability is postponed and compressed into fewer years at the end of life."

We will die after approximately a few minutes without oxygen, one week without water, or a month without food, but it might take thirty years for lack of exercise to kill us. The effect is the same. It just takes longer.

The pearl in the sometimes rough shell of exercise is the abundant joy and vitality that come from doing it regularly. Exercise doesn't just save your life—it makes you feel good, too. The key is to try to find something you enjoy.

We believe that physical fitness has five components: cardiovascular endurance, muscular strength and endurance, balance and agility, flexibility, and body composition. Healthy levels of these components can be achieved through a wide variety of activities. It is up to you to find things you like and experiment with different types of exercise.

Here are some key tips:

### Begin a habit of regular aerobic or cardiovascular exercise

If you're a beginner, try walking—even just five minutes a day is a good start.

Build up slowly to at least thirty minutes a day, four days a week, of vigorous aerobic exercise. Any time of the day is fine, as long as it's at least two hours before bed.

Use a heart rate monitor to check your heart rate during exercise, or learn how to take your pulse in your neck or wrist. (You can feel your pulse just below the pointy part of the angle of your jaw—count your pulse for fifteen seconds and multiply by four.) Getting a cardiometabolic stress test, or even a regular stress test, can help give you a more accurate range and a better exercise prescription. Ask your doctor.

Try to get in and stay in your target heart rate during your workout. As mentioned, a rough way to figure your maximum heart rate is to subtract your age from 220. If you're fifty, your maximum heart rate is 170. Your target heart rate is between 70 and 85 percent of your maximum heart rate. Thus if your maximum is 170, your target is 119 to 144.

Experiment with different forms of exercise: walking, swimming, jogging, roller-skating, jumping rope, rowing, cycling, spinning, exercise machines, cross-country skiing, skating, kick boxing, dancing, bouncing on a mini-trampoline, or hiking a mountain. Try water aerobics—it's easy on the joints and is especially recommended for pregnant women. Or dancing—put great music on and rock away!

Be sure to increase your level of exertion as your fitness level improves. If you stay at the same speed and incline on the treadmill for years without increasing your effort, your benefits will go downhill.

### Begin a gradual strength-training program to build muscle and stamina

Just twenty minutes three times a week can be enough to stop the otherwise inevitable muscle loss of ten ounces a year that affects most of us over forty. It can prevent the "skinny-fat syndrome," that all-too-familiar phenomenon of weighing the same at age sixty as at twenty, but having twice as much fat. Your muscle has been replaced by fat, with all the related dangerous consequences, but you still can fit into the same clothes.

Try anything that builds strength. Besides weights, consider calisthenics, Dynabands (stretchy bands you can take with you anywhere), or even power yoga or Pilates, a system of core strengthening.

Be careful to start slowly and with proper supervision. Hurt comes easily when you first start exercising. Sometimes your muscles are not strong enough to protect your joints, ligaments, and tendons from injury. If you can afford it, hire an experienced, well-recommended trainer for those first few weeks. Guidance can be critical. Not only might you otherwise miss the benefits of exercise, you may harm yourself if you don't use machines or free weights properly.

If you try strength training, build up to two sets of eight to twelve repetitions for each of the four major muscle groups (chest and shoulders, upper back, upper legs, and abdominals) three times a week. This should take you about twenty minutes for each session, or an hour a week.

### Start a daily yoga practice or stretching routine

We get stiffer as we age, but it is never too late to become flexible. As excellent as it is, exercise shortens muscle fibers and contracts muscles. Stretching balances out this process, preventing injury and reducing pain overall.

Yoga is a wonderful system of stretching that engages the whole body. Its combination of stretching and careful breathing offers a powerful overall effect that can also reduce stress and calm the nervous system. Find a yoga class, or get a yoga tape, CD, or video; they come in many styles and experience levels.

Keep in mind: Never force your body to do what it doesn't want to. If you hurt, ease up. You will get further by breathing and relaxing into a pose than forcing yourself into it.

If you don't enjoy yoga, consider basic stretching routines. Just a few minutes of stretching a day can go a long way to improving your health. But be careful of trainers who do the stretching for you—these people may mean well, but they can cause harm when they ignore your whimpers of pain, or worse, tell you that you need to be stronger and love the pain. "No pain, no gain," they say, but the truth is, that pain may well be telling you something important, such as, "Stop right now!"

Take a class at the gym, or buy a book and stretch at home. You can even close your office door and do a set of stretches there that will make sitting behind a desk that much easier.

### Maintain a healthy body composition

The ideal body percentage for fat for a man is 10 to 20 percent of his weight; for a woman it is 20 to 30 percent.

Remember, you can be overfat, or underlean, even if you are not overweight. The skinny-fat syndrome is a sure route to rapid aging and disease.

You can monitor your body composition with calipers or DEXA body composition techniques. Calipers are available at many gyms or sport facilities. The DEXA body composition gauge is the gold standard, but is usually found only at hospitals or through exercise physiologists.

### Assess and treat the body's structural problems

Repairing our body isn't just about exercise. Just as problems with our internal organs and biology can affect our outer structure, structural problems in the body can affect our internal functioning.

Our structure and function must both be working well for us to be healthy. Many of us have injuries, or have experienced traumas, or simply have sat at our desks or in front of our computer monitors or televisions for too long. Sometimes, problems come simply from carrying a heavy briefcase with the same arm over and over. In some way, most of us become a little lopsided.

Over time, these minor problems can put stress on our bodies that leads to breakdown and dysfunction. If an area is restricted in any way, the blood flow is reduced to that area, and the body can't repair it well. The tissues lack oxygen, and damage occurs that starts a cascade of oxidative stress, inflammation, and pain.

These problems have solutions. Aches and pains you thought you had to live with forever may disappear as you learn new patterns of movement. Many therapies and techniques are available for regaining structural balance and physical integrity. Here are some suggestions to start with:

Consider assessment and treatment by an osteopath, cranial osteopath, chiropractor, physical therapist, myofascial therapist, or other qualified body worker to manage chronic physical imbalances.

Find a good physiatrist (a doctor who specializes in rehabilitation or physical medicine) to identify problems and prescribe corrective therapies.

Consider regular body work such as massage, deep tissue massage, Rolfing, neuromuscular therapy, myofascial release, Thai massage, or shiatsu.

Try movement therapy techniques, including Feldenkrais, Alexander Technique and Somatic Education, Qi Gong, Tai Qi, and Trager. All of these are designed to help with the restoration of full movement and function to your body, and to release old physical and emotional traumas stored within it.

### 3. PRACTICE STRESS MANAGEMENT

Stress is defined as a real or imagined threat to your body or your ego. Being chased by a tiger has the same biological effects as feeling oppressed by your boss.

Our daily routine does little to invoke the body's best healing forces. When we try to do five things at once and feel incapable of completing any of them, we stew in our own stress juices—cortisol, glucose, insulin, adrenaline, free radicals, inflammatory proteins, and more.

That wouldn't be quite so bad if we were able to discharge those chemicals. Ever wonder why you feel calm and relaxed after a good workout? You may be running on a treadmill rather than running from a saber-toothed tiger, but the effects are the same. You burn off those harmful stress chemicals.

Well-known author and researcher Hans Selye discovered the stress response by accident. Selye was an absentminded lab scientist whose rats were always escaping from their cages and then being chased. When Selye later examined these rats, he found their thymus (immune) glands had shrunk and their adrenal (or stress) glands had enlarged. In other words, the stress of escape and capture had changed the rats' internal chemistry.

Prolonged and unrelieved stress contributes to or causes a staggering amount of illness. Yet just as exercise trains the body and helps it adapt to stresses, specific habits and techniques must be practiced to strength our relaxation "muscle." We must all find and press our "pause buttons."

Following are some suggestions that can provide an antidote to stress, and help achieve powerful healing in the process. Simply practicing these recommendations will go to the heart of the five forces of illness. The chemical reactions set in motion by these behaviors will help nourish you, reduce inflammation and oxidative stress, and improve detoxification and metabolism.

### Honor your limitations
Know the limits of what you can do in a day. Remember that true multitasking is for computers, not people.

### Learn that you cannot please everyone all the time
In fact, if you try, you will likely not please yourself.

### Take mini-vacations throughout the day
Close your eyes in your chair at work for ten minutes, breathe deeply, and think about a beautiful place that can restore your soul.

### Try meditation

It doesn't matter which religion or lifestyle you borrow it from. Anything that can calm you down is helpful. Here's a Buddhist meditation that we like—try saying it to yourself whenever you want to take a moment's vacation:

> *Breathing in, I breathe in the world's pain.*
> *Breathing out, I send it healing love.*
> *May all beings be happy.*
> *May all beings be peaceful.*
> *May all beings be kind.*
> *May all beings be free.*

### Learn to breathe well

Restricted or shallow breathing prevents oxygen from reaching all of your tissues and can profoundly affect your energy and lead to stress. Proper breathing is a quick route to healing and relaxation. It can be done anywhere, at any time of the day, even in short bursts. Breathing deeply and fully will oxygenate your brain, body, and spirit, transforming your health in the process.

Try the following exercises. For each, close your eyes and, if possible, sit or lie in a comfortable position on your bed, in a chair, or on the floor (on a pillow).

Belly breathe: Put your hand on your belly. Breathe out, squeezing the air out of your lungs with your stomach muscles. As you breathe in, relax your stomach muscles and, after filling your lungs, try to push your hand off your belly with your breath, filling the lower part of your lungs. Continue to breathe in and out slowly through your nose. Each in and out breath should last to the count of three. Do this for five minutes a day, or whenever you feel stressed.

Observe your breath: Simply notice the breath coming in and out of your nostrils for five minutes a day. Keep your mouth closed and pay attention to the rhythm of your breath.

Count your breath: Breathe in slowly through your nose to the count of four. Breathe out even more slowly to the count of eight. Do this for five minutes anytime during the day.

### Learn and practice the art of doing nothing

Just as farmers let fields go fallow to regenerate the land, doing nothing is actually doing something. It is a time to reset your internal rhythms, to integrate the experiences of the day, to be directionless. It is a place where creativity and happiness begin. It's also harder to do than you might think! We have run into patients who say that spending an hour dedicated to doing nothing is more difficult than getting five tasks done at once. Try it and see if you're good at nothing.

### Try progressive muscle relaxation

Many well-studied and proven techniques exist for turning on the relaxation response and counteracting the effects of stress. For example, try progressive muscle relaxation: Tense and hold a major muscle group for ten seconds, relax for five seconds, then move on to the next muscle group. Start with your facial muscles, then your neck, shoulders, each arm, buttocks, each leg, and each foot. Notice how this makes you feel.

### Consider support groups or psychotherapy

A great deal of research has shown the positive effects of social support in terms of reducing infection, cancer, heart disease, and other ailments. Simply joining something as simple as a bowling group can have a salutary effect.

### Listen to music

Sounds and music can affect your physiology and biochemistry directly. In one study of cardiac patients, listening to ocean sounds and symphonic music for thirty minutes caused a reduction in blood pressure, respiratory rate, and psychological distress. Research has shown that music may influence central physiological variables, including blood pressure, heart rate, respiration, EEG measurements, and body temperature. Music also influences immune and endocrine function. Listen to any music that makes you feel good, use soothing music at night before bed, or listen to Dr. Andrew Weil's *Sound Body, Sound Mind: Music for Healing.*

### Find any way to relax that works

Take a walk in the woods, romp around with your dog or cat, play a game with a friend—all of us find joy and peace and restoration in different activities. Find those that work for you and pen (not pencil) them into your schedule. They are not optional for good health.

### Don't worry

Worry can be fatal. Studies show that anxiety increases your risk of a heart attack by three to seven times. In most cases, worry produces few results other than making us ill.

Worry is a habit and can be unlearned, although it isn't easy. Like exercising an atrophied muscle, it may be painful or difficult at first, but with practice and help (meditation, yoga, psychotherapy, breathing, and so on) you can strengthen the emotional and psychic muscles that can help keep you healthy and happy.

## 4. PRACTICE OTHER ULTRAPREVENTION TECHNIQUES

### Find meaning and purpose

The art of creating purpose in our lives may look different for each one of us, but whatever we do, however we decide to live our lives, the meaning we extract from our work and our relationships plays a large part in determining whether we thrive and age well, or become ill and die young.

A remarkable study published in the *Journal of the American Med-*

*ical Association* radically challenged our common notions about why there has been an increase in illness in the segment of our population with less education and less income. In the past, research attributed this trend to bad habits, including poor diet, lack of exercise, smoking, alcohol consumption, and obesity. But the new study found that even improving health behaviors in the disadvantaged would not correct the discrepancy in death and disease.

Instead, the major factors seemed to be a dearth of social relationships and support, as well as personality issues such as lack of optimism, sense of control, and self-esteem; high levels of anger and hostility; and chronic and acute stress in life and work.

Seeking to infuse meaning into your life can go a long way toward preventing illness and death and increasing vitality and health. We realize this is much easier to say than to do, but it's impossible to avoid a discussion of the above with any patient. Good physical health does not exist in a vacuum, and no doctor can truly know his or her patients without understanding their inner lives. We often suspect that no matter how good a person's physical health, without an accompanying sense of deeper purpose in life, really good, long-lasting health is difficult to attain.

### Build healthy relationships and social connections

Endless research shows us that a rich social network of friends and family is critical to good health. In some cases, the effect may even be powerful enough to help us overcome bad habits.

Researchers from Temple University studied the health of an immigrant Italian population in Roseto, Pennsylvania, and found that their rich social connections, the collective celebration of family passages and religious festivals, and the sense of community felt by the residents were associated with a 50 percent reduction in deaths from heart attacks, despite the fact that the residents tended to smoke, eat rich diets, and didn't exercise.

Another study, in Alameda, California, found that close social ties, marriage, and belonging to a religious or community organization had profound effects on lessening the risk of death from cancer, heart disease, and stroke. The most socially isolated individuals had more than three times the risk of death compared with the socially connected.

The extent of your social connections can even influence the number of colds you get each year. In one study, each of 276 volunteers had rhinoviruses (the common cold) dripped into their nose. Those with the fewest social connections had four times the chance of actually getting colds.

Here are just a few ideas to get you thinking:

• Call a family member daily just to say "I love you."
• Make dates with your friends at least once a week, even if just for tea, or make late-night phone calls.
• Invite friends over for a meal. You don't have to be a cook to do this. Make it a potluck dinner. Just provide a nice atmosphere for friends to share food and conversation.
• Join a support group—it doesn't even matter what kind. If you feel as though you don't have enough people to talk to, a support group can give you an instant circle of listeners.
• Volunteer in your community. Volunteering is not only a wonderful gift of time and energy, it helps you feel good about yourself.
• Contact a church, temple, community agency, relief fund—there are many outlets just waiting for you to call.

### Keep a journal

Writing down your thoughts and feelings can have a powerful effect on your psyche, as well as on your immune and nervous systems. In a study published in the journal *Clinical Psychology* (February 1998), therapeutic writing was shown to have significant physiological effects, including many beneficial changes such as better skin conductance, increased helper and suppressor lymphocyte function (white blood cells that fight cancer and infection), and reduced levels of cortisol, as well as psychological improvements such as greater well-being and better social functioning, and behavioral improvements such as raised grade-point averages and fewer visits to the doctor.

In another recent study published in the *Journal of the American Medical Association,* seventy-one patients with asthma or rheumatoid arthritis were asked to write about various aspects of stress over a period of days; the study showed a significant improvement in standard measures of disease severity in both conditions four months later.

Buy a journal or create a private file on your computer to record your feelings and thoughts. Take twenty minutes three times a week to write about your life's most stressful events. When you have finished with all those (and for some of us, that can take years), start writing about the most stressful events of your current week.

### Consider therapy

There are many times when we have told patients that they might want to consider some form of psychological therapy. We don't do this as a dark threat but as a way of guiding people toward another form of health support.

Psychotherapy has proven effective in treating and preventing many different illnesses, from heart disease to cancer to chronic fatigue. Seek counseling or psychotherapy in any of its forms, although we personally favor cognitive therapy, which can help to activate your healing system.

Consider seeking out a counselor, whether you're recovering from illness, or simply feel the need to work out issues that might otherwise reveal themselves through your health.

### Schedule play

We often feel sad when we talk to our hardworking patients who have spent a lifetime providing for their families and find that they don't know how to stop working. They have forgotten how to play.

Play takes practice. It doesn't happen by itself, and playfulness is the secret source of vitality that children access every moment. Play is great therapy. Cultivate playfulness in your everyday life. Take dancing lessons. Make a snowman. Roll down a hill with a kid. Do something every day with no other goal than to enjoy yourself. Have fun! It's good for your health.

That's it! That's the six-week plan. You now have all the information you need to stop falling for all the myths of modern medicine. And you have all the information you need to start a new, healthy life.

As we said, this will take some work on your part. But why wouldn't you want to make good health your goal? And why would you want to depend on a doctor who has only a few minutes to listen to you, who is bound by a system that hinders rather than helps, and who probably knows less than you do about your health?

A wise healer once said about the medical practice, "If you listen carefully to your patients, they will tell you exactly what the problem is."

As marvelous as modern medicine is, no one has ever invented anything better than the simple act of listening. That requires time, however, something medicine has taken away from the modern physician, whose model is to talk for a few minutes, and then scurry to form a diagnosis, recommend a specialist, and order expensive tests—or maybe all three.

If listening is old, and also the foundation of what we call our new medicine, what makes ultraprevention so new?

It's because we have new questions to ask and new ways to listen to the answers. Ultraprevention is a set of glasses to view the world through, a pair with lenses significantly different from those used fifty years ago. Back then, medicine was simpler; the main concerns included maternal and infant mortality, and infectious diseases such as pneumonia, tuberculosis, and smallpox. Many of these afflictions have now all but disappeared. Modern advances in maternal and infant health, nutrition, immunizations, hygiene, and the treatment of infectious diseases have dramatically improved human life in the past century.

We are now entering an age in which we are able to envision medicine not simply as a remedy for ailments, but as a tool to realize our true human potential. Instead of viewing medicine as a system to diagnose and treat conditions, we are achieving the luxury of using medicine to allow us all to live our lives to their very fullest. This is the ultimate aim of ultraprevention, and it's hard to imagine a more empowering goal.

# ACKNOWLEDGMENTS

**MARK HYMAN:**

My life's circuitous journey has provided me with many teachers, including my professor of Zen at Cornell, Dr. Alan Grappard, who helped me see that things were not always as they appeared, and who taught me how to ask the best questions to find the best answers. I also want to thank all the professors at medical school who answered "because" to my continual question "but why," and who inflamed my passion to understand the nature of things. I must especially thank Jeffrey Bland, Ph.D., a true genius and truly noble man who selflessly created the Institute for Functional Medicine, where physicians can learn the skills needed to practice the future of medicine today.

Medicine is a maturing science; I am standing on the shoulders of the great scientists, thinkers, and physicians of the last two hundred years, yet I am also standing on the shoulders of lesser-known but often more powerful men and women of compassion and vision; without their help I would not have been able to see the incredible vista of medicine in front of me. This list is endless, but I must thank my personal mentors and teachers, Sidney Baker, M.D., Leo Galland, M.D., Andrew Weil, M.D., Dean Ornish, M.D., David Perlmutter, M.D., Michael Lyon, M.D., and Bethany Hays, M.D. And I thank my closest friends, Marc David and David Piver, who helped me find the truth and follow it to the most unlikely places. They asked me "why" and never settled for "because." And, finally, thanks to my past and my future, Pier.

**MARK LIPONIS:**

I would foremost like to thank each and every one of my patients for teaching me and helping me to become a better physician. I would also like to thank my mentors and advisers who have both taught and inspired me—Alan Michelson, M.D., James Dalen, M.D., Andrew Weil, M.D., and Dr. Jeffrey Bland.

Both of us would like to thank all of our patients from our years of practice, as well as all of our colleagues at Canyon Ranch, especially Dr. Cindy Geyer; Dr. Nina Molin; Dr. Stephanie Beling; Kathie Swift, Canyon Ranch's extraordinary nutrition director; and the nutrition staff, who first taught us that fat is not a four-letter word. We would also like to give our thanks to the entire health and healing professional and support staff.

We must especially acknowledge the ever-generous and thoughtful owners of Canyon Ranch, Mel and Enid Zuckerman, whose foresight and tenacity made their wonderful vision a reality, and Jerry Cohen, Canyon Ranch's excellent CEO. We thank them for having such faith in us and for giving us the unparalleled opportunity to practice medicine in a setting where we could dive deeply into the world of our patients.

And we would like to thank our new friends in the publishing business, especially our warm and wonderful editors, Tracy Behar and Beth Wareham, whose enthusiasm for this project has never waned. Our agent, Richard Pine, has also been unfailing in his support, and we will always be grateful to him for all he has done. We are very lucky to have found these consummate professionals.

Finally, we are inestimably indebted to our cowriter, Gene Stone, who has patiently guided us through the publishing process from start to finish. We are aware that doctors aren't always the easiest of collaborators, but even when the going was tough, Gene always made sure that the project never flagged. His ability to bring out the best in each of us is startling. He has been more than a collaborator. He has been a friend.

# INDEX

## ABOUT THE AUTHORS

**Mark Hyman, M.D.,** and **Mark Liponis, M.D.,** are co–medical directors of Canyon Ranch, a practice affiliated with Harvard University's Brigham and Women's Hospital. They share conventional medical educations, backgrounds as general practitioners in poor, rural communities, and are both survivors of catastrophic illnesses, which led to their strong commitment to holistic, health-based medicine.